THE
ATKINS
ESSENTIALS

Also by Robert C. Atkins, M.D.

Atkins for Life
Dr. Atkins' New Carbohydrate Gram Counter
Dr. Atkins' Age-Defying Diet
Dr. Atkins' Vita-Nutrient Solution:
Nature's Answer to Drugs
Dr. Atkins' Quick & Easy New Diet Cookbook
Dr. Atkins' New Diet Cookbook
Dr. Atkins' New Diet Revolution
Dr. Atkins' Health Revolution
Dr. Atkins' Nutrition Breakthrough
Dr. Atkins' Nutrition SuperEnergy Diet Cookbook
Dr. Atkins' SuperEnergy Diet
Dr. Atkins' Diet Cookbook
Dr. Atkins' Diet Revolution

Coming Soon in Paperback
The Atkins Shopping Guide
by Atkins Health & Medical Information Services

Coming Soon in Hardcover
Atkins Diabetes Revolution
by Robert C. Atkins, M.D.

THE
ATKINS
ESSENTIALS

A TWO-WEEK PROGRAM TO JUMP-START
YOUR LOW CARB LIFESTYLE

 ATKINS HEALTH & MEDICAL INFORMATION SERVICES

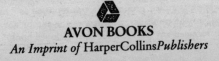

AVON BOOKS
An Imprint of HarperCollinsPublishers

The information presented in this work is in no way intended as medical advice or as a substitute for medical counseling. The information should be used in conjunction with the guidance and care of your physician. Consult your physician before beginning this program as you would with any weight-loss or weight-maintenance program. Your physician should be aware of all medical conditions that you may have as well as the medications and supplements you are taking. Those of you on diuretics or diabetes medications should proceed only under a doctor's supervision. As with any plan, the weight-loss phases of this nutritional plan should not be used by patients on dialysis or by pregnant or nursing women.

AVON BOOKS
An Imprint of HarperCollins*Publishers*
10 East 53rd Street
New York, New York 10022-5299

Copyright © 2004 by Atkins Nutritionals, Inc.
ISBN: 0-06-059838-7
www.avonbooks.com

First Avon Books paperback printing: January 2004

Avon Trademark Reg. U.S. Pat. Off. and in Other Countries, Marca Registrada, Hecho en U.S.A.
HarperCollins® is a registered trademark of HarperCollins Publishers Inc.

Printed in the U.S.A.

10 9 8 7 6 5

➤ Acknowledgments

This new book, the first one published since the death of Dr. Atkins, was written by the team at Atkins Health & Medical Information Services and carries on his legacy of providing practical nutritional information to help people enjoy healthier lives. Although he did not live to see this book published, we are certain that Dr. Atkins would have been proud of its objective—to make the Atkins Nutritional Approach™ accessible to everyone.

Michael Bernstein, senior vice president of Atkins Health & Medical Information Services, manages the group's efforts to continually offer information and educational materials directly to people, with the hope that through understanding the truth about Atkins, more and more people can manage their weight and improve their health. Editorial director Olivia Bell Buehl oversaw the development of this book and as usual was supported by a superb team of trained professionals. Managing editor Christine Senft, who is also a nutritionist, gave the project her usual care and attention. Food editor Stephanie Nathanson worked tirelessly to make the food sections crystal clear for Atkins beginners and organized the meal plans, collaborating with recipe developers Wendy Kalen and Cynthia DePersio.

Nutritionist Colette Heimowitz, M.S., director of education and research for Atkins Health & Medical Information Services, wrote the introduction and provided overall guidance. Jacqueline Eberstein, R.N., director of education, who worked with Dr. Atkins for almost 30 years and with him helped thousands of patients lose weight and improve their health, reviewed the manuscript for accuracy and made many helpful suggestions. Nutritionist Eva Katz, M.P.H., R.D., compiled the research studies validating the Atkins program.

Three writers who contribute regularly to the Web site *www.atkins.com* and to other Atkins publications were key in getting *The Atkins Essentials* from concept to the book you hold in your hands. Health expert Lynn Prowitt-Smith produced much of the manuscript, with valuable contributions from medical writer Sheila Buff and food writer Martha Schuenemann.

The team at Morrow/Avon pulled out all the stops to get this book done in record time. Editor Sarah Durand suggested the basic idea for the book, and then applied all her editorial skills to help make it as useful and well organized as possible. Special thanks to Michael Morrison, Libby Jordan, Kristen Green, Anne Marie Spagnuolo, Elizabeth Glover, Juliette Shapland, Jeremy Cesarec, and everyone at Morrow/Avon.

Contents

► Introduction

If you're reading this, it's likely that you or someone you care about needs to lose weight. So first, bravo to you for wanting to do something about it! The latest national figures are truly depressing: According to a 2002 article in the *New England Journal of Medicine*, more than 64 percent of Americans are overweight and more than 30 percent qualify as obese. Both figures are up significantly since the 1990s. According to the National Institute of Health, approximately 280,000 Americans die each year of causes related to obesity. And it's not only heart disease and diabetes—as a person's weight increases, so does the risk of dying from cancer.

Since millions of people have slimmed down, gotten on the road to good health and changed their lives as a result of the Atkins Nutritional Approach™ (ANA), you're holding the right book in your hands. After 40 years of experience, we feel it is safe to say that the ANA is the most successful approach to weight loss in existence. If you follow the instructions in this book— to the letter—you, like the vast majority of other people who have done Atkins, will experience amazing success in losing weight and feeling better than you ever have before.

In a nutshell, doing Atkins is based upon the concept that your body burns both carbohydrates and fat for fuel. Cut back significantly on carbohydrate foods like pasta, bread and potatoes, as well as sugar, and your body burns fat, including its own fat, for fuel. The result is that you lose weight.

This book is by no means a substitute for *Dr. Atkins' New Diet Revolution*. Consider this an essential supplement to that ANA classic. We found that many people were looking for a quick guide to Atkins—something that would help them get started on the original low carb lifestyle ASAP without necessarily delving into the physiological explanations of carbohydrate metabolism. Maybe you're one of those people. When you're ready to do something, you don't always want to take the time to read the whole manual before you start. So think of this book like the quick set-up guide you get when you buy a new computer. *The Atkins Essentials* will tell you how to plug in, turn on and get started!

To continue the analogy, remember too that it's extremely important to eventually sit down and read through the whole computer manual—because it gives you a much fuller understanding of how to make the best use of your machine. Once you've experienced initial success doing Atkins, you'll be eager for the more detailed information you'll need to maintain that engine (your body) and to troubleshoot in case you encounter a barrier down the road. Similarly, you'll want to take the time to read *New Diet Revolution* later so you'll have a broad knowledge of your new controlled carbohydrate lifestyle as well as an in-depth look at the future phases of the ANA. And when you are homing in on your goal weight, *Atkins for Life* will help you maintain your newly slim body and enhanced health.

This book is divided into five sections. First you will quickly learn the advantages of doing Atkins, and then you'll move on to the vital chapters that usher in your new lifestyle. Part Three focuses on the all-important subjects of eating and cooking, complete with two weeks of meal plans and a handful of delicious recipes suitable for the first phase of Atkins, Induction. Part Four gives you a basic understanding of the three phases that follow Induction and outlines a healthy way of eating that will last you a lifetime. Part Five includes more than 100 of the most frequently asked questions—and answers—about doing Atkins. We also provide a glossary of terms and an abbreviated list of research studies that support the principles upon which the ANA is based.

What this book will do for you:

- Jump-start your weight loss
- Prepare you for a new lifestyle
- Walk you step by step through the first two weeks
- Help you troubleshoot any individual concerns
- Answer the most frequently asked questions about doing Atkins

- Provide complete meal plans and recipes for your first two weeks
- Introduce you to the three, more liberal, phases of Atkins that follow Induction
- Convince you once and for all that exercise is essential to good health and weight control
- Encourage you to learn more about the Atkins lifestyle by visiting *www.atkins.com* and by reading *Dr. Atkins' New Diet Revolution* and *Atkins for Life.*

We want to stress again that although this book focuses primarily on the first two weeks of the Atkins program, controlled carbohydrate eating is not a quick-fix approach to weight loss. Nor is Induction the same as the ANA. Sad but true, unless you are willing to commit to eating the controlled carb way for the rest of your life, you will almost certainly gain back any weight you lose.

That said, you're in for many delightful surprises. Doing Atkins allows you to indulge in the most satisfying, luxurious, delectable foods—all while improving your blood pressure, cholesterol and overall health. Oh, and let's not forget the mirror. Just wait until you slide into those jeans and get a good look at the slimmer, healthier and more attractive you!

Colette Heimowitz, M.S.
Director of Education and Research
Atkins Health & Medical Information Services

PART ONE

Why Atkins?

1 ➤ What You'll Gain from Doing Atkins

Before I started doing Atkins, I was 60 pounds overweight and had high blood pressure, high cholesterol, and severe headaches. I decided to try Atkins. Within just a few days, my energy level increased and I was enjoying foods that not only tasted good but also filled me up. After about eight weeks, I had lost 40 pounds, my total cholesterol had dropped from 520 to 173 and my triglycerides went from 740 to 119. Six weeks later, my tests were even better. Because I was feeling so good, I decided to take up running and eventually ran a marathon! Today, I am 60 pounds lighter, my blood work continues to be excellent, and my headaches are practically gone. It's been two years since I started my program, and I like myself a lot more today than I used to. Both my energy level and my outlook are much improved, and not just because I'm thinner, but because I'm healthier.

—Brendan Adams, lost 60 pounds

You already know what you'll lose on Atkins—weight. But do you have any idea how much you have to gain? You are in for a wonderful ride. While the pounds drop off, you'll reap dozens of other fringe benefits as a result of making the switch to a controlled carbohydrate lifestyle. Some of these benefits come right away, during your first two weeks of the first phase, called Induction. Others come later and will truly change your life. So let's first take a look at the benefits you'll begin enjoying during the first two weeks on the Atkins Nutritional Approach™ (ANA).

► Immediate Return on Investment

1. **Lose weight without counting calories.** Although you do need to count grams of carbohydrate on Atkins—at least until you get close to your goal weight—this is nowhere nearly as painful as counting calories. Of course, you can lose weight by limiting the calories you eat, but the problem is that most of us end up hungry all the time—and feel weak and miserable as well—on a low calorie diet. And after you've lost weight this way, it almost inevitably creeps back on, because very, very few people can bear to be hungry—and grumpy—forever. In contrast, when you do Atkins, you can eat all the calories you need to feel satisfied—and the fat on your abdomen, hips, thighs and wherever else it is lurking will melt away. And since you're not hungry, weak and miserable eating this way—on the contrary,

you'll feel satisfied and full of energy—you'll be able to stay with the program and keep the weight off. That's why we regard Atkins as a lifestyle, not a diet that you go off once you've shed some weight.

WHAT ARE CARBS?

Most people think of carbohydrates only as sugars and starches such as in rice and potatoes; however, all fruits, vegetables, and grains contain carbohydrates. Other foods, such as cheese or legumes (kidney beans and their kin) contain carbohydrates along with fat and/or protein.

---

2. **Control your cravings; curb your appetite.** As you will learn in this book, carbohydrates turn into glucose, or sugar, when they're absorbed into your blood. When you eat something like a jelly doughnut, which contains a high dose of carbohydrates, it results in a sudden rise in the amount of sugar entering your bloodstream. This rise is followed by a big dip, as your body chemistry tries to adjust. When those dips occur, your body sends an urgent message to your brain: Get me more sugar! When you do Atkins and stay away from nutrient-deficient, carb-laden foods, however, your blood sugar remains relatively stable throughout the day. This means no more of the food cravings or false hunger pangs that result from those sudden blood sugar dips.

WHAT ARE "BAD" CARBS?

The carbohydrate foods you want to eliminate from your diet forever are breads and pasta made from bleached flour, foods full of sugar in all its forms (including honey and high fructose corn syrup) and convenience foods and snacks (junk foods). Highly processed and low in nutrients, these "bad" carb foods put you on the blood sugar roller coaster.

WHAT ARE "GOOD" CARBS?

During the Induction phase of Atkins, your carbs will come mostly from salad greens, plus dozens of other vegetables such as asparagus, broccoli, green beans and cauliflower. Atkins Nutritionals, Inc. has developed many low carb foods that are also suitable for this phase. These carbohydrate foods are full of nutrients, as are the carb foods you will eventually add back into your regimen in later phases of the program: seeds and nuts, berries, whole grains, legumes, other fruits and even small portions of starchy vegetables such as sweet potatoes.

3. **Enjoy wholesome, nutrient-dense foods.** Another reason you won't be plagued by hunger when you do Atkins is the quality of the food you'll be eating.

That means, bite for bite, you're consuming more of the nutrients your body needs than you do when you eat the high carb, processed foods that make up so much of the typical American diet. If you stop feeding your body empty calories, or "fillers"—such as crackers, cookies, bagels, pasta and sugary drinks—and instead provide it with highly nutritious foods, you'll feel satisfied sooner, and that satisfaction will last longer. The bonus? At the end of the day, you may end up eating less food without even trying.

4. **Savor "luxury" foods.** You've probably gone through much of your life believing that to be thin and healthy, you need to avoid rich foods like shellfish, butter, cheese, mayonnaise and cream. You've probably heard people say, "I'm being bad," because they're eating bacon and eggs. Maybe you've said it yourself. When you do Atkins, being "good" is no longer related to depriving yourself of all the most delicious foods. You can eat filet mignon with béarnaise sauce, scallops sautéed in butter, and cheese omelets. When everyone else is asking for vinaigrette dressing on the side or half a lemon, you can order blue cheese or creamy ranch! You can have hollandaise, cream cheese and whipped cream—virtually all of your formerly forbidden "fattening" foods.

5. **Get fast results.** Nothing helps you stay focused on a new eating plan more than seeing the pounds—and inches—come off. When doing Atkins, most

people see a significant, exhilarating drop in their weight during the first two weeks. Some of this is water, as is the case when you start any weight-loss program. If you are someone who tends to retain fluid and often feels bloated or puffy, you'll enjoy this side benefit; Atkins is an effective diuretic. The rest of what you lose, however, will be fat. In just a few days after beginning Induction, you will begin to burn your body's fat for fuel.

6. **Get your appetite under control.** Once your body makes the shift from burning carbohydrates to burning fat, you will also notice that your hunger pangs dissipate. You may even—hold onto your seat—*forget to eat*! (As you will learn later on, even if you are not hungry at mealtimes, you should have a small snack so you don't find yourself ravenous a few hours later.) At the same time, you will likely feel your energy level skyrocket. You'll also find that your mood improves, you'll rid yourself of addictions to caffeine and/or sugar and you'll even find that your newly stable blood sugar means that you'll sleep more soundly. All this in the first two weeks! And the best news of all, it just keeps getting better.

These are just some of the immediate benefits you'll enjoy in your first weeks doing Atkins. And you'll be setting a great example for your children as you improve your diet and health.

As you continue on your new eating plan, you're in

for more good news. You probably know that losing weight alone has a direct benefit on your health, reducing your risk for a myriad of conditions, including high blood sugar, high blood pressure (hypertension), diabetes, cardiovascular disease and even certain types of cancer, and dramatically improving the quality of your day-to-day life. (People with arthritis and joint diseases also report improvements in their symptoms.) However, you may not know that losing weight by switching to a controlled carbohydrate eating program brings with it a host of additional health benefits.

Kicking all that sugar and white flour out of your life does a body good—a lot of good. By making Atkins your permanent lifestyle, you will:

- Decrease your risk for heart disease
- Prevent, forestall or control diabetes
- Lower your blood pressure (if it is high)
- Prevent or alleviate many other health conditions

You'll be pleased to know that these benefits are scientifically proven facts. For a listing of hundreds of research studies that support the principles upon which the ANA is based, go to The Science Behind Atkins, at *www.atkins.com*.

Now let's look closer at these long-term health improvements.

▶ **What Atkins Does for Your Future**

1. **Decreases your risk of heart disease.** This one may surprise you because so many of us were taught that eating fat—which you must do on Atkins—raises cholesterol and, therefore, the chance of developing heart disease. The truth is that if you do Atkins correctly, meaning that you eat only healthy natural (that is, untreated) fats without also eating lots of carbohydrates, you are bound to reduce your risk for this country's number-one killer disease. If you look at the biggest risk factors for heart disease, you'll find that doing Atkins positively affects almost all of them. On Atkins, you are very likely to:

   - Lose weight
   - Lower your total cholesterol
   - Raise your good (HDL) cholesterol
   - Lower your triglycerides
   - Lower your blood pressure if it is high
   - Stabilize your blood sugar and insulin levels

   If you read that list out loud to a physician, he or she would say you've just provided a prescription for heart disease prevention. That is exactly what Atkins can do for you, along with reducing your risk for developing diabetes and other conditions related to abnormal blood sugar and insulin levels. Remember, before he became an expert on weight control, Dr. Atkins was a cardiologist.

When my doctor told me I had diabetes, I was shocked. I was very overweight but I was only 32 years old! To the astonishment of my doctor, coworkers and family, going on Atkins helped bring my blood sugar level into a normal range without medication. As a wonderful side effect, I lost 99 pounds!

—April Greer, lost 99 pounds

2. **Prevents or controls diabetes.** Type 2 diabetes is a disease caused by years of blood sugar (and insulin) run amok. Unlike Type 1 diabetes, in which the body produces insufficient insulin, with Type 2 diabetes, the body's fat cells resist the action of insulin. In healthy individuals, insulin transports the excess blood sugar to the cells. But for Type 2 diabetics, too much sugar remains in their bloodstream. This disease occurs when someone has a genetic predisposition to it, eats a diet filled with refined carbohydrates, or lives a sedentary lifestyle—or, often, a combination of all three things. Most people with diabetes are overweight or obese and have been overconsuming carbohydrates for years. And here's a frightening statistic: According to the American Diabetes Association, 17 million people—a full 6.2 percent of the population—had diabetes in the year 2000. Of these, 11.1 million were diagnosed. That means that a staggering 5.9 million, or one third of the total, are undiagnosed and unaware that they have this life-threatening condition.

If you've decided to do Atkins because you have been diagnosed with Type 2 diabetes, you'll find that moderating your carb intake will put you in control of your blood sugar level. Many diabetic people find that they can eventually reduce or discontinue their medications if they follow the Atkins program. **(Important: Never stop or reduce the dosage of any medications, including insulin or other diabetes medications, without your doctor's supervision.)** And if you are doing Atkins to kick your carb addiction, lose weight and improve your health, you may very well be unknowingly putting the brakes on an inevitable descent into diabetes. The bottom line: The ANA is a lifestyle that is defined by its ability to lower and control abnormal blood sugar. Whether or not you have a strong family history of diabetes, you may well be able to stall or completely avoid its onset by sticking to a controlled carbohydrate lifestyle. Many of the damaging effects of abnormal blood sugar (and insulin) levels occur silently prior to the actual diagnosis of diabetes. Prevention is essential.

Weight loss is just one of the benefits I've experienced since going on Atkins. The stiffness and strains in my back and neck have disappeared. My cholesterol and triglycerides are lower. Overall, I just feel like a healthier person. I even get fewer colds!

—James Winterscheid, lost 122 pounds

THE CONNECTION BETWEEN
BLOOD SUGAR, INSULIN AND DIABETES

When you eat carbohydrates, which increase the sugar in your bloodstream, your pancreas produces insulin to transport the glucose to cells for energy or fat for storage. Over time, excessive carbohydrate consumption (and the resulting insulin production) means that it takes more and more insulin to keep your blood sugar level normal. Over time, your pancreas runs out of insulin, which ultimately leads to diabetes. In the simplest terms, diabetes is the inability of the body to keep blood sugar at a normal level.

3. **Lowers your blood pressure.** Hypertension, or high blood pressure, often goes hand in hand with unstable blood sugar and being overweight. If you have one of these conditions, it's likely that you also have or soon will have the other. Doing Atkins helps bring blood pressure under control in two ways. First, losing weight alone is one of the most effective ways to lower high blood pressure. But if you lose weight the Atkins way, by cutting down on carbohydrates, you'll be normalizing blood sugar (and insulin) levels, which are likely connected to your elevated blood pressure. And if you're among the people with high blood pressure who are also sensitive to salt, Atkins will arm you with one more defense. Getting your blood sugar and insulin under

control will also reduce fluid retention, helping lower blood pressure yet another way.

Like many women, my weight problem started after I had children. By the time my daughter got married, I weighed 216 pounds and had developed high blood pressure. I started Atkins and lost 12 pounds in the first week. I thought to myself, "Wow, there's a person in there." Eight weeks later, my blood pressure had already dropped. I had so much energy and strength it amazed me. Seven months later, I had lost a total of 70 pounds. And I am now confident I can maintain my healthy weight. People can eat anything in front of me and I'm not bothered.

—*Barbara Woodruff, lost 70 pounds*

4. **Prevents or alleviates other health problems.** We have been amazed over the years at how many different types of health problems significantly improve when people do Atkins. Many digestive complaints, such as severe heartburn, the development of gallstones, gas and bloating improve significantly when people switch to a controlled carbohydrate lifestyle. (Some people experience constipation during the first phase of Atkins, but supplementing with fiber until you are consuming fruits and more vegetables in the later phases should

alleviate this. See "Coping with Constipation" beginning on page 96.)

Another condition that often improves markedly in women who do Atkins is polycystic ovarian syndrome (PCOS), a hormonal imbalance that can cause irregular menstruation, infertility, weight gain, acne, excess body and facial hair, high insulin levels and even symptoms of diabetes. An estimated 6 to 10 percent of all women between the ages of 20 and 40 have this syndrome. The exact mechanisms of PCOS are not well understood and there is no cure, but in his 40-year practice, Dr. Atkins consistently observed that a controlled carbohydrate lifestyle helped many of his patients keep their symptoms under control and avoid long-term complications.

Finally, people who switch to Atkins often report that a host of other physical ailments seem to have magically disappeared. Problems such as insomnia, chronic headaches, migraines, sinus problems, abdominal pains, acid reflux, asthma, eczema, acne and other rashes abate and then go away altogether. It's very likely that food allergies or food sensitivities are involved in many of these cases. Most of the foods that commonly provoke allergic reactions are high carbohydrate foods such as corn, wheat, oats, sugar or milk.

It can be very difficult to isolate a food allergy or sensitivity while eating the typical American diet. Doing Atkins makes it easy to separate out these foods, as you only reintroduce high carbohydrate

foods into your meals in the later phases of the plan—
and then only in small amounts, one at a time—so
any negative reaction will be obvious.

Not only do Atkins followers find themselves suffering less from their aches, pains, heartburn and
rashes, but they end up taking a lot less medication
when they work with their physician to decrease
dosages or eliminate certain drugs. This means sav-
ing money, but more important, it means that you
can avoid the regular bodily assault of all those
drugs and their side effects, which in some cases include weight gain. (We'll talk more about how certain medications can interfere with weight loss in
Chapter 7.)

Now that we've covered the short- and long-term
benefits of Atkins, you may be wondering, "Why isn't
everyone following a controlled carbohydrate eating
plan?" It is clearly the healthiest way to eat. As you've
now heard, the human body reacts extremely well
when you stop feeding it a high carbohydrate, highly
processed-food diet. One reason everyone doesn't eat
this way is that the giant food companies have a vested
interest in continuing to produce and create new products made from wheat, corn, sugar and other inexpensive and highly refined carbohydrates. (Just imagine
what it would be like to go to a supermarket and find
none of these products filling aisle after aisle!)

Another reason is that the old myths and misconceptions about Atkins and controlled carb eating still cir-
culate, even among highly educated people and

professional health care practitioners. Old ways of thinking persist even after scientific study after study reveals that Atkins is as effective or more effective than low fat programs in both weight reduction and reduction of risk factors for disease. Once you've lost your unwanted pounds and see how good you feel eating this way, you'll probably want to spread the word and correct some of the misconceptions people have. In Chapter 3, we'll give you all the information you need to help set the record straight about this healthy, life-changing way of eating.

But first, in the next chapter, we're going to look at why this program works. It's not magic, even though it sometimes seems that way to people who have been waging war against their own excess weight for years, tried diet after diet and seen lost pounds vanish only to return with a vengeance as soon as they go off each successive diet. When you get a handle on the nuts and bolts of eating excessive carbohydrates and what they do inside your body, you'll see that it's simple and logical—not hocus-pocus at all.

► Food for Thought

This chapter has probably got you contemplating your eating history, your overall health, the way you feel each day—things you may not have thought a lot about before now. To get the most out of this book, take a few minutes at the end of Chapters 1–9 and make some notes to yourself. We'll provide the questions to get you rolling, and you take it from there. You can use a notebook or keep a journal on your computer. This exercise will help you solidify your commitment to your new way of eating—and living.

What are your personal health issues? Do you have a family history of heart disease, diabetes or hypertension? Are your cholesterol or triglyceride levels high?

_____

_____

_____

_____

_____

_____

Do you get heartburn, gas or bloating? Other digestive problems?

_____

_____

_____

Do you think you might unknowingly suffer from a food sensitivity or allergy?

_____

_____

_____

Do you get mysterious headaches, pains or rashes?

_____

_____

_____

How many over-the-counter and prescription medications do you use for non–life-threatening ailments? Have you ever read the package inserts in their entirety?

_____

_____

_____

How is your energy level? Do you have definite highs and lows each day?

_____

_____

_____

How well do you sleep? How many hours does your body seem to need? Do you wake up feeling refreshed and energetic?

_____

_____

_____

Think about a typical pre-Atkins day of eating for you. How much refined white (bleached) flour (often listed as "enriched wheat flour") do you consume? Don't forget to include anything with breading or batter, any white pasta and any baked goods. And how much sugar (often listed as "corn syrup or high fructose corn syrup") do you consume every day? Remember, there's hidden sugar everywhere—in your bread, crackers and bagel; and in your dressings, sauces and condiments—and even in such over-the-counter medications as cough syrups.

_____

_____

_____

Do you crave certain foods and are you unable to control those cravings?

_____

_____

Are you sleepy after meals?

_____

_____

Do you have symptoms that are relieved by eating?

_____

_____

_____

2 ► Why Atkins Works

My history includes heart problems, hospitalizations and a morbidly obese body that topped out at 465 pounds when I was 40. But I'll tell my story to anyone who will listen, because it's a miracle. Atkins enabled me to shed 240 pounds. Once I had to take a laundry list of prescription heart medications and painkillers. Today, I take none. Before, it was a challenge to walk across the room and my health problems prevented me from holding down a job. Now my wife and I have our own thriving business.

—George Stella, lost 240 pounds

You may already be convinced that Atkins works. You probably know of people who have lost significant amounts of weight and improved their lives as a result of doing Atkins. And now you've read a few more real-life accounts and heard about the incredible benefits that come from adopting this new lifestyle. Still, we want you to have the whole picture and to fully understand the basic logic behind Atkins. So let's have a quick Nutrition 101 overview of what exactly is in the food we eat.

▶ What's in Your Food?

Everything you eat is made up of some combination of three key components, called macronutrients, that supply the calories our bodies need to function: **protein, fat** and **carbohydrate**. Depending on the food, it also contains varying amounts of water, fiber, minerals, vitamins, phytochemicals, antioxidants and other nutrients.

Protein is essential for building and maintaining your muscles, bones, organs and other tissues and to keep your body functioning. Meat, fish, poultry, eggs, cheese and other animal foods are known as complete proteins, meaning they have all of the essential amino acids for building and repairing your body and its systems. Nuts, seeds, legumes (beans, including soy products such as bean curd, or tofu) and whole grains contain protein but they don't have all the necessary essential amino acids. This means they need to pair up with other foods to form a complete protein.

Fat comes in a few different forms—some of it very good for you and some of it very bad for you. Dietary fat is important for vital body functions such as making hormones, building cell walls and storing energy. Fat comes from meat, fish, poultry, dairy products, nuts, seeds, and their oils, and even a few vegetables and fruits and their oils—such as olives and avocados. The only truly bad kind of fat—despite what you've heard repeatedly in our fat-phobic culture—is called trans fat, or trans fatty acids. This kind of treated fat is found in most processed foods, listed in the ingredients as hydrogenated or partially hydrogenated vegetable, corn, soy, coconut or palm oil. Even though this oil comes from natural foods such as soybeans or corn, the chemical process known as hydrogenation turns it from a good, or neutral, thing to a very bad thing.

Typically, Americans get too much trans fat and too much of the common vegetable oils like corn oil and safflower oil and not enough of the fats that come from fish, nuts, seeds and avocados. It's best to consume a balance of natural, unprocessed fats in both food and supplements. In terms of bottled oils, this means choosing "cold-pressed" or "expeller-pressed" oils, such as olive oil and flaxseed oil.

Carbohydrate includes sugars and starches. Carbohydrates provide the quickest source of energy and, especially in the form of vegetables, contain a wide variety of vitamins and minerals, enzymes and fiber. Carbohydrates can be either unrefined or refined. Unrefined carbohydrates occur in vegetables, fruits and whole grains. Refined carbohydrates are contained in products not found in nature, the ubiquitous examples being sugar, corn syrup and pasta, white rice and flour. Like hydrogenated oils, these carbs start off in nature as harmless foods, but when they are processed, synthesized or altered in the manufacturing process with chemicals, they turn into blood sugar spiking substances. The refining process strips the carbs of their health-promoting substances. The change in the American diet over the last century from one in which the carbohydrates consumed were primarily in the form of vegetables, fruits and whole grains to one in which most carbohydrates are processed flour, sugar, and products made from these and other refined carbohydrates is partly responsible for the nation's epidemics of obesity and diabetes.

Carbohydrates are sometimes classified as simple and complex. In general, simple carbohydrates are sugars such as sucrose (table sugar) and fructose (the sugar in fruits), lactose (sugar in milk), and maltose (sugar in malt). Complex carbohydrates are found in all vegetables, grains and legumes. But the distinction between simple and complex is misleading. That's because when your body digests complex carbs, including starches such as grains, it breaks them down into simple carbs at a slower rate—but in the end, all complex carbs are converted to simple carbs. This explains why you need to control your consumption of complex carbohydrate foods such as corn and potatoes. An exception to this rule is fiber: It is one class of complex carbohydrate that your body cannot digest, making it a valuable ally in appetite control—and therefore weight management—by giving you a feeling of fullness. It also aids in "cleansing" your digestive system.

➤ A Closer Look at Carbs

Now that you've completed Part One of our very condensed Nutrition 101 course, you probably want to know how you go about controlling your intake of the food components that are not good for your body. The good news is that when you do Atkins you can partake of a wide variety of proteins and fats as long as you are eating until you are satisfied but not gorging yourself. Doing Atkins is all about eating whole foods. The crux of the matter is in limiting carbohydrates and in selecting the right carbohydrates, those most full of nutrients and fiber and those with the lowest impact on your blood sugar.

Since carbohydrate foods include all the fruits, vegetables, grains and starches on the planet, you do need to know exactly what to eat to control your carb intake. (Foods such as milk, cheese, nuts and legumes also contain carbohydrates along with fat or protein or both.) Atkins followers control the number of grams of healthy carbohydrates they eat, while making proteins and fats the centerpieces of their diets in the initial weight-loss phases. Not only is it important on Atkins to choose foods with low carb counts, it is also crucial to select the most nutrient-dense carbohydrate foods.

VEGETABLES

Vegetables, in general, contain "good" carbohydrates, although some are very high in carbs and not as high in nutrient value, and some are the reverse. Most vegetables provide fiber and many healthy phytonutrients (*phyto* means "plant"), those magical substances found in plants that help us ward off disease. Despite what you may have heard, the Atkins Nutritional Approach™ (ANA) prescribes a greater amount of vegetables than the average American eats. Fortunately, the vegetables that are most dense in nutrients happen also to be those lowest in carbs. Salad greens and other leafy greens eaten raw—Boston and romaine lettuce, escarole, spinach, parsley, watercress, arugula—are all nutrient powerhouses that are also low in carbs. Other excellent choices include asparagus, bamboo shoots, broccoli, cabbage, cauliflower, collard greens, eggplant, jicama, kale, kohlrabi, leeks, mustard greens, okra, onions, pumpkin, radishes, scallions, shallots, snow pea pods, spaghetti squash, string or wax beans, Swiss chard, tomatoes, turnips, water chestnuts and zucchini (a complete list of acceptable Induction foods begins on page 75).

During the first phase of Atkins, in which carbohydrates are most limited, you can eat three cups of low carb vegetables daily. Depending on your personal preference, you can choose to have two cups of salad vegetables and one cup of the other type (broccoli, eggplant, snow peas, spinach, etc.) or three cups of salad vegetables. During the increasingly liberal phases that follow, you will add more and more vegetables. By the final phase, called Lifetime Maintenance, most people can eat every kind of vegetable, although the higher carb/lower-nutrient ones should always be eaten in moderation or only rarely.

FRUITS

Although most fruits do fall into the category of "good" carbohydrates, they contain the most sugar of all whole foods and are not allowed during the first phase of Atkins, which lasts a minimum of two weeks. However, because they are rich in phytonutrients and fiber, some of them can be reintroduced in the second phase, called Ongoing Weight Loss, and you can increase the amount you eat in each subsequent phase of the ANA. (We'll look at the three phases that follow Induction in greater detail in Part Four.)

The first type of fruit allowed is berries, which have the lowest carb count and the highest nutrient punch of any fruit. After berries, other relatively low carb and high nutrient fruits include apples, cherries, grapefruit, peaches, pears, plums, oranges and tangerines. The highest carb fruits include bananas, mangoes, prunes and raisins. Fruit juices, too, are very high in sugar and they lack the fiber that you get in whole fruit—they should be avoided or consumed in small quantities only when you are at or close to your goal weight.

Tip: One way to enjoy fruit juices in later phases of Atkins without overdosing on carbs is to dilute them with mineral water.

GRAINS

Grains are very high in carbohydrates and are only allowed in the later phases of Atkins. This category includes corn, whole wheat, brown and wild rice and oats, as well as all wheat flours and pastas. Once you are approaching your goal weight and are completely in control of your food choices, you can reintroduce whole, unprocessed grains into your diet. You will always want to keep your portions small and you must avoid the refined grains found in most mass-market products. If you're not familiar with whole grains, it's worth educating yourself when the time comes. Head to the natural foods store: There's a whole world of nutrient-rich textures and flavors out there—and whole grains are very filling, so it's easy to keep your portions small. Increasingly, well-stocked supermarkets also are selling these and other healthy alternative foods.

Until three years ago, I bought into the low fat idea. I'd use fat-free cooking spray. I ate bagels, bread, pasta and piles of white rice. At breakfast, I used low-cal, fat-free syrup on my pancakes. I thought I was doing everything right. But I couldn't lose weight and I felt lousy. I would fall asleep after carb-laden meals and often felt drowsy at work. When I started Atkins, I felt better right away and soon the weight started falling off. And my doctor was amazed at how much my cholesterol had improved. The best, though, was when someone pointed me out recently as "the skinny guy!"

—*Mark Anthony Monticule, lost 30 pounds*

► **The Blood Sugar Roller Coaster**

Now that you understand what carbohydrates are and which foods contain high amounts, it's time to address the question of why they cause problems when consumed in excess. In Chapter 1, we talked a bit about carbohydrates and blood chemistry and how sugar cravings occur. Here, we'll delve in a bit deeper.

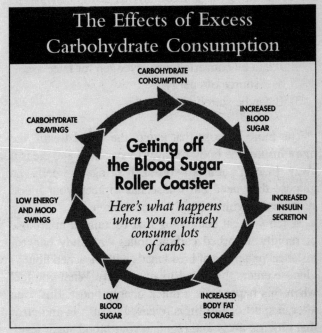

The Effects of Excess Carbohydrate Consumption

Getting off the Blood Sugar Roller Coaster

Here's what happens when you routinely consume lots of carbs

- CARBOHYDRATE CONSUMPTION
- INCREASED BLOOD SUGAR
- INCREASED INSULIN SECRETION
- INCREASED BODY FAT STORAGE
- LOW BLOOD SUGAR
- LOW ENERGY AND MOOD SWINGS
- CARBOHYDRATE CRAVINGS

When you eat foods that contain carbohydrates, they impact your blood sugar levels. This is because all carbohydrates are converted into glucose, or sugar, when

they reach your bloodstream. The amount of carbs—
and the type—will determine the degree of impact. For
example, a food full of sugar and bleached flour such
as a sweetened breakfast cereal will raise blood sugar
much more dramatically than does a green salad.

Once the glucose is delivered to your blood, it has to
be transported to your cells to do its work. The hormone insulin is the carrier that transports glucose to
the cells. Once the glucose arrives at the cells, three
things can happen to it:

1. It can be used for immediate energy.
2. It can be converted into glycogen for later use
   as a source of energy.
3. It can be stored as fat.

The more glucose that enters the bloodstream, the
more insulin the body releases to sweep in and clear it
away. Insulin's job is twofold: It brings the cells the
glucose they need but it also has to keep your blood
sugar levels within a fairly normal range.

When you eat something that contains a high dose
of rapidly absorbed carbohydrates—a candy bar, for
instance, or a piece of bread made with bleached flour—
glucose enters the bloodstream quickly. What you feel
when this happens is a quick energy boost. But soon
after, a spurt of insulin is released to rush in and clear
that glucose away and regulate your blood sugar level.
Because your body wasn't designed to deal with candy
bars and refined flour, it digests them so rapidly the insulin response may overshoot its mark, clearing away

too much of the glucose. This results in a drop in blood sugar, which leads to an energy crash—what many people experience as the afternoon slump. It becomes hard to concentrate or you may feel downright lethargic or sleepy. You're likely to find yourself craving some chocolate or potato chips or anything packed with carbs to get that blood sugar soaring again. And so the roller-coaster ride continues.

On the other hand, when you eat foods that are mostly protein or fat, your body produces far less insulin and these extremes in blood sugar are avoided. (We should note here, however, that if you gorge yourself on protein, some of it can be converted to glucose. But even excess protein does not have the same effect as refined carbohydrates.) When you produce less insulin, your blood sugar level remains constant and along with it, your energy level. Eating this way gets you off the blood sugar roller coaster and on to the smooth-riding energy train.

▶ Insulin: The Fat Hormone

As we just mentioned, insulin transports glucose to the cells and drops it off first to the cells that need it for immediate energy. If the cells already have plenty of glucose for fast energy, the excess is turned into glycogen, which is stored in the liver and muscles, where it is readily available for later use. However, once all the glycogen storage areas are filled—and we have only a limited capacity for storage—the body has to do something with the leftover glucose. And when you think about how much carbohydrate most Americans consume each day—and how little energy they expend—you know we're talking about significant amounts of leftover glucose. Here's what happens: The liver converts the remaining glucose to fat, which becomes the stores of jiggly body fat on your belly, thighs, buttocks and elsewhere. That's why insulin is known as the fat hormone. Think about all those people walking around out there who still think it's *fat* that makes them fat! Now you know better: *Excess carbohydrates are the true culprit.*

▷ What Are Net Carbs?

There's one last thing you need to know about carbohydrates. On Atkins, you count **Net Carbs**, which represent the total carbohydrate content of a food *minus* its fiber content. You can subtract those grams of fiber because they are a type of carbohydrate that doesn't significantly impact your blood sugar level. As you can guess, this gives you an incentive to pick high-fiber foods—which, nutritionally speaking, are almost always a healthy choice.

Fiber not only has a neutral effect on blood sugar, it also does quite a bit of good in other ways. Fiber slows digestion, which in turn slows the conversion of carbs into glucose headed for your bloodstream. It is also valuable in keeping hunger at bay. That's because fiber is bulky and absorbs water, so it fills you up quickly and makes you feel full longer. And, of course, fiber's benefit for regularity is well known.

In packaged foods, you can look at the nutritional information label and do the math, because the carbohydrate and fiber contents will be listed in grams. However, you won't be eating much in the way of packaged foods (other than all the Atkins low carb convenience foods suitable for Induction listed on page 84), so you'll have to rely on a carb counter. *Dr. Atkins' New Carbohydrate Gram Counter* (M. Evans) is a handy pocket-size booklet, or go to *www.atkins.com* and use the online carb counter found under the Food & Recipes tab.

GO AHEAD, YOU DO THE MATH!

Here's the simple formula for determining Net Carbs for any food:

Example: 1 whole artichoke
13.4 grams **Total Carbohydrate** – 6.5 grams **Fiber** = 6.9 grams **Net Carbs**

Down the road, in the later phases of Atkins, you'll be able to explore more of the hundreds of new, delicious low carb products that have come on the market in recent years, thanks to the explosion of interest in controlled carbohydrate eating. You'll see other carbohydrate ingredients listed on these products that, like fiber, have minimal impact on blood sugar and don't

Nutrition Facts

Serving Size 1/2 Cup (56g)
Servings Per Container 6

Amount Per Serving

Calories 210   Calories from Fat 35

	% Daily Value*
Total Fat 3g	**5%**
Saturated Fat 0.5g	**3%**
Cholesterol 0mg	**0%**
Sodium 280mg	**11%**
Total Carbohydrate 13g	**5%**
Dietary Fiber 8g	**33%**
Sugars 2g	
Protein 29g	**58%**

Vitamin A 0%	•	Vitamin C 0%	
Calcium 8%	•	Iron 20%	
Thiamine 4%	•	Riboflavin 0%	
Niacin 4%	•	Folate 2%	

*Percent Daily Values are based on a 2,000 calorie diet. Your daily values may be higher or lower depending on your calorie needs:

	Calories:	2,000	2,500
Total Fat	Less than	65g	80g
Sat Fat	Less than	20g	25g
Cholesterol	Less than	300mg	300mg
Sodium	Less than	2,400mg	2,400mg
Total Carbohydrate		300g	375g
Dietary Fiber		25g	30g
Protein		50g	60g

Calories per gram:
Fat 9 • Carbohydrate 4 • Protein 4

*For those controlling their carbs, count only 5 grams of the 13 grams of the Total Carbs in this product. Subtract dietary fiber (8g) which has a minimal impact on blood sugar.
Learn more: www.atkins.com/netcarbs

have to be counted. These include glycerine and sugar alcohols.

That's the end of your abridged Nutrition 101 course and our brief look at the science of carbohydrates. You're almost ready to begin doing Atkins. We'll spend the next chapter telling you a few things you should do before starting, putting to rest any lingering doubts or questions you may have about the ANA and giving you answers to all the questions you'll get from those friends, family members and coworkers who aren't yet in the know.

▶ Food for Thought

If you've been trying to lose weight for some time, you may have come to consider yourself an expert on food and nutrition. However, this chapter may have given you pause, providing you with new information about your body and its reaction to the foods you eat. Use these questions to evaluate your current eating behavior and how it makes you feel.

What are your favorite protein foods? What are some dishes made with those foods that you really love?

_____

_____

_____

_____

_____

_____

_____

What high fat foods have you typically tried to avoid in the past? What are your favorites? How about whipped cream, brie cheese, olives, avocados, chicken complete with skin, salmon and red meat? (Forget fried foods breaded with flour and/or bread crumbs.)

_____

_____

_____

In your current way of eating, where does most of your dietary fat come from? Were you aware of the dangers of hydrogenated vegetable oils?

_____

_____

_____

Do you routinely check ingredient labels? Do you know how to read the data presented? Do you always check serving size?

_____

_____

_____

When you read about some of the vegetables that have low carb counts, which jumped out at you? Are there some that you've never tried or, perhaps, never heard of? Do you think you'll enjoy trying some of these new vegetables? (All you have to do is wash them, steam or sauté them and put on a little butter or olive oil!)

_____

_____

_____

Have you ever been aware of a blood sugar "crash" after eating a very high carb meal or snack? Do you get frequent cravings where you can't stop thinking about a certain sugary food you know is in your kitchen or desk drawer? Do you find it hard to have just one bite of certain high carb foods?

_____

_____

_____

Did you used to think that eating fat made you fat?

_____

_____

_____

3 ▶ Getting Ready to Do Atkins

I had been heavy most of my life and had tried unsuccessfully to diet. When I graduated from college, I weighed 240 pounds. I heard about Atkins from someone at work and decided to read Dr. Atkins' New Diet Revolution. *It seemed written just for me and made so much sense. Over the course of a year, I lost 90 pounds and have maintained my weight for more than a year and a half. I've had to put up with a lot of naysayers. My friends, coworkers and family members all told me that eating this way would make me sick. I am happy to say that they were all wrong and I am the healthiest and happiest I've been in my life!*

—Amy Wright, lost 90 pounds

Although controlling your carbs will be a cinch once you've gotten used to it, the first week or two can be difficult. You and your body are making a big and sudden

switch and it takes a little time to adapt. The best thing
you can do to ensure success is to prepare properly. That
includes readying your kitchen, your loved ones and
even your own mindset. It definitely means consulting
with your doctor. Overall, you want to anticipate any
challenges you may face so that nothing stands in the
way of a smooth transition to your new lifestyle.

▶ Before You Begin . . .

1. **Clear your schedule.** Ideally, your first 14 days, or
   at least the first seven days of doing Atkins, should
   take place during one of the calms amid life's
   storms. Look at your calendar and find a lull. This
   should be a period when not much is happening in
   your life. For example, you are better off not starting when you're embarking on vacation, traveling
   for business, entertaining, going to parties or eating
   out a lot. It's not that you can't do Induction while
   doing all these other things. It's just that it will be
   much harder to stay focused and eat only what's on
   the "Acceptable Induction Foods" list (see Chapter
   5). After you're through the first two weeks and are
   firmly into fat-burning mode and have established
   your new routine, you will find it much easier to
   travel and pursue an active social life.

   On the other hand, if your schedule is always de-
   manding and you want to move forward, by all
   means go ahead. As Dr. Atkins used to say, "Just
   give me two weeks."

2. **Give friends and family a heads up.** For some, the hardest part of making a life change is dealing with the people around you. Sometimes friends and family express concern because they don't want to see you disappointed, especially if you have struggled with your weight for a long time and tried out a variety of diets. Other times, even those nearest and dearest to you might feel threatened when you start to make changes in your life. You may no longer fit conveniently into the category they have put you in, or your new mindset may threaten their image of themselves. Whatever their motivations, if family or friends weigh in with conflicting advice, you've got to be diplomatic but firm. Tell people that this is important to you and you would appreciate their support—or at the very least, keeping their opinions to themselves. (See "From Sabotage to Support" on pages 44–45.) This should be a problem only at the beginning: Once your loved ones begin to see the results, you'll find that you no longer need to defend your choices.

If you don't live alone, prepare the people who live with you by explaining your new eating style to them. If you are the primary cook, just make a protein dish and vegetables and prepare a few additions for those who are not following Atkins. You may have to suffer a little temptation, but if you really want to lose weight you'll have to bite the bullet. If someone else does the cooking, explain exactly what you can and cannot eat. If your "cook" is willing, have him or her read Chapter 5.

3. **Get your food in order.** Have your kitchen well stocked with the foods you can eat so you'll never find yourself going hungry. You'll want to have foods around that you can grab quickly if hunger overtakes you. Prepare foods to have at the ready, such as tuna salad, hard-boiled eggs and sliced chicken breast, and keep olives, avocados and cheese on hand. (See "Stocking Your Kitchen," beginning on page 162, for other ideas.) It is also convenient to stash some low carb bars or ready-to-drink shakes in your office, purse or car, in case hunger strikes or if a meal is delayed. Having such foods within reach will help you ignore the temptations of the coffee cart or the fast-food joint you pass on your way home from work.

Just as important, if you live alone, get rid of the things you're not allowed to eat. If you have a family or housemates, try to dedicate one cupboard and section of the fridge to the foods you *can* eat so that you don't have to confront "forbidden" foods every time you open the refrigerator or cabinet.

4. **Stock up on the recommended nutritional supplements.** A key component of doing Atkins is supplementing with a quality multivitamin/mineral and essential fatty acids.

5. **Measure up.** Before you begin doing Atkins, hop on the scale and record the number. Getting the truth, no matter how much you hate admitting it, down in black and white is an important part of your commitment to change. Also use a tape measure to

measure your chest, waist, hips, upper arms and thighs, and record these numbers as well. When you measure yourself a week later and then again in two weeks, you'll be happy you did. The more ways you have of gauging your success, the more encouraged you'll be.

6. **Start a food diary.** Keeping a journal can be an invaluable partner in helping you reach your goals. By charting what you eat from day to day, you'll begin to see the patterns that contribute to your success, as well as retrace your steps when you've temporarily gone astray. It will also help you see if certain foods are getting in the way of your journey to a slimmer, healthier you. You'll get to know your eating habits, identify nutritional stumbling blocks and explore emotions and other lifestyle issues that may have a bearing on your relationship with food. Finally, having a private place in which to record your emotions can help you stay motivated about making changes in your life.

7. **Come up with an exercise plan.** Exercise is an essential part of doing Atkins. You may not want to implement this plan, however, until after the first few days on Atkins. In the first 48 or 72 hours, you may feel tired and a bit off-kilter as you shift your body's metabolism to burning fat as its primary fuel. Be sure to check with your physician before starting to exercise if you have been inactive or are stepping up your pace of exercise.

FROM SABOTAGE TO SUPPORT

Here's how to deal with well-meaning friends who wittingly or unwittingly try to undermine your weight-loss goals: When you announce to your friends and family that you're planning to lose weight by doing Atkins, chances are good that at least someone in that group is going to try to talk you out of it. These are people who are important to you, but they're attacking your decision. How can you turn them from saboteurs into supporters? Here's a guide to reading the real meaning behind your friends' words and how to reply to them.

What They Say, What They Mean

The first step is to see beyond the things these people say to the unspoken reasons for their lack of support. Once you understand their hidden or unconscious motives, you'll be able to respond in a way that helps them understand and respect your decision. Take these examples:

What they say: You look fine as you are.
What they mean: If you are no longer the same overweight person I already know, it will shake things up and make me uncomfortable.
What you reply: I know I need to lose weight to improve how I feel and how I look. I'm determined to do this. I think I deserve your support.

What they say: Nobody can stick with the Atkins approach—it's too restrictive.

What they mean: You haven't stuck to any other diets. Why should I think you'll stick with Atkins?

What you reply: I've looked into it carefully, and everything I've learned convinces me that Atkins is easier to stick to than low fat, low calorie diets.

What they say: You've gone off every other weight-loss program you've ever tried. Why bother with yet another one?

What they mean: Here we go again—now I have to hear all about yet another diet that doesn't work in the end. I'm getting tired of being supportive and then seeing you be let down.

What you reply: Yes, I've failed to lose weight (or maintain weight loss), but I'm committed to success this time. If you can't support me in my decision, at least don't undermine me.

What they say: Doing Atkins is bad for your health.

What they mean: I've heard a lot of half-truths and misinformation about Atkins.

What you reply: I've researched Atkins and read a lot about it, and there's just no evidence to what you say. To prove it, why don't you read *The Atkins Essentials* or *Dr. Atkins' New Diet Revolution* for yourself, or check out the Why Atkins Works section of *www.atkins.com*?

FINDING THE SUPPORT YOU NEED

Change is never easy, even when you're doing Atkins. It's even harder when the people around you aren't being very supportive. There will inevitably be times when you're tempted to fall back into the trap of your old eating patterns, so you need someone who understands how you feel and can encourage you to stay on plan. Sometimes that person can be a sympathetic family member, a good friend or an Atkins buddy. Many husbands and wives find that doing Atkins together draws them closer and helps them hang in for the long term. When one is tempted to cheat, the other can remind him or her of the long-term goals and vice versa. Siblings or friends can provide the same kind of support.

If you are not in a relationship or your significant other is not interested in doing Atkins, you may want to find an online Atkins buddy through one of the many Web sites dedicated to controlled carb weight loss. The Atkins Web site (*www.atkins.com*) includes a section called My Atkins that helps you chart your progress and provides support. Another excellent source for online support for doing Atkins is *www.ediets.com*.

If you can't get support from the people around you, another route is to find it in the help of a professional counselor or therapist. Even when you have a good support network, a professional can help you gain insight into the complex emotional issues behind overeating. Although a professional therapist can be expensive, some of the cost may be covered by your health insurance. You may also be able to find skilled low-cost or even free support through your local community health system.

▶ Medical Support

There is one very important thing you should do before you start Atkins or any weight-loss program: See your physician. Schedule an appointment to get a complete physical, including blood work, to test your cholesterol and triglyceride levels, and other clinical tests. It's important to have a medical workup before beginning Atkins, both from a health perspective and to help motivate you to follow the program faithfully. A physical may uncover a health problem, such as prediabetes, that you were not aware of and that may make doing Atkins all the more vital.

You also should stop taking any nonessential over-the-counter medications, such as cough syrup or cough drops containing sugar. Many prescription medications also inhibit weight loss. Talk to your doctor to see if you can find alternatives.

In addition, there are several categories of drugs that can cause adverse effects when taken while on a controlled carbohydrate eating plan. First are the diuretics, because reducing your carbohydrate intake alone can have a dramatic diuretic effect.

Second, since Atkins is so effective at lowering high blood sugar, people who take insulin or oral diabetes medications can end up with dangerously low blood sugar levels.

Third, Atkins has a strong blood-pressure-lowering effect and can easily convert blood-pressure medications into an overdose. If you are currently taking any of these medications, you will need your doctor's help to adjust your dosages.

Be sure your doctor measures your lipid levels, which will reveal your total cholesterol, HDL ("good") and LDL ("bad") cholesterol and triglycerides. These indicators often change when you alter your diet. Blood chemistries will measure your glucose (blood sugar) and your kidney and liver functions. Your doctor also should measure your uric acid levels. Since some people mistakenly believe these indicators are negatively affected by doing Atkins, you may later regret not having a "before" baseline to compare with your "after" results three months after starting Atkins. For more details on all these tests, see *Dr. Atkins' New Diet Revolution*.

Don't wait to have your initial lab work done until *after* you start Atkins, because then you may think any abnormalities are the result of your new way of eating. You may well have had even higher cholesterol and triglycerides before you began.

Your doctor also will check your blood pressure. High blood pressure and being overweight often go together. Having high blood pressure (also called hypertension) puts you at clear risk for stroke and heart disease and may indicate elevated insulin levels. What happens to high blood pressure on Atkins? It goes down. Nothing is more consistently or more rapidly observed than normalization of blood pressure.

Note: People with severe kidney disease should not do any phase of Atkins, unless approved by their physician. Moreover, the first three phases of Atkins are not appropriate for pregnant women and nursing mothers. They may safely follow the Lifetime Maintenance phase, but should not do Induction or any of the other weight-loss phases of Atkins.

TALKING TO YOUR DOCTOR ABOUT ATKINS

More and more physicians are clued into Atkins and support their patients' decision to follow a controlled carb approach to weight control. In case your doctor is not, here's how to bring him or her up to speed:

- **Be proactive.** It's up to you as the patient to provide the evidence to overcome any objections your doctor may have. See "Dispelling the Myths," pages 51–58, for a list of the misconceptions about Atkins that still prevail and how you can respond if your physician raises any of them.

- **Provide the backup.** Once you've cleared up any misconceptions about doing Atkins, it's time to provide your doctor with some solid scientific studies that support its underlying principles. There are far too many of these to give a complete list here, but ask your doctor to check out the particularly important studies listed on pages 349–352. For more studies, visit The Science Behind Atkins, at *www.atkins.com*.

- **Make a deal.** The best way to overcome any objections raised by your physician may not be with research, but with results. Tell him or her that you'll do Atkins for three months, and at the end of that time, you'll come in for another checkup. When your doctor sees that in that short time you've lost weight, improved your blood cholesterol and triglycerides, brought your blood pressure down and that overall you're feeling more energetic and positive, you'll have made your point.

➤ Resolve Your Own Questions

Because the Atkins way of eating is diametrically opposed to the mainstream mantra we've been spoonfed for years (low fat, low fat, low fat!), it has been the subject of furious debate since the publication of *Dr. Atkins' Diet Revolution* 32 years ago. Dr. Atkins developed—and continued to refine—what is now called the Atkins Nutritional Approach™ (ANA) based on his observations over 40 years of working with tens of thousands of patients.

In the last three years, there have been numerous research studies conducted at prestigious universities and hospitals that validate the efficacy and safety of the ANA. Repeatedly, these research papers published in peer-reviewed medical and nutritional journals have demonstrated that controlling carbohydrate intake for weight loss is as effective—and usually more so—than cutting fat and calories. Moreover, these same studies have shown significant improvements in markers for cardiovascular health when individuals follow Atkins or other low carb regimens. If you have any lingering doubts about the route on which you are about to embark, you may want to review some of these studies. (See pages 349–352 for a representative list. A complete listing is available at *www.atkins.com.*)

► **Dispelling the Myths**

Despite an ever-increasing body of research, opinions change slowly. You may have heard negative things about Atkins from friends or relatives or the media, even health professionals who are not aware of this validating research. There are still many myths and misconceptions about Atkins, even as the supportive research accumulates and experts and practitioners finally come around. It takes years for a major paradigm shift in nutritional dogma to take hold, however. In the meantime, while we wait for the "trickle down" of new information in the mainstream media, we'll set the record straight here in order to put to rest nagging doubts standing in the way of your full commitment to doing Atkins. Moreover, we want you to feel confident explaining to others why and how the ANA is the healthiest way to eat and that it is supported by solid research.

The first and perhaps most important perspective to realize is that the food you eat when you do Atkins is surprisingly close to what our primitive ancestors ate. Meat, fish and poultry; nuts, seeds and berries; vegetables and salad greens—the caveman would have recognized most of those things. (Although you do not eat seeds and nuts during the first two weeks of Induction, they are one of the first foods you add, as are berries.) But they wouldn't have known what to make of all those boxes filled with sugar, white flour and processed foods lining the aisles of your supermarket. When you consider that evolutionary changes in the human body take eons to occur (think of wisdom teeth or tailbones), it's logical to assume that our physiology is still best suited to a diet similar to that of our ancestors. Our bodies certainly haven't made the switch to thriving on processed, sweetened carbohydrates—our epidemics of obesity and diabetes make that painfully clear.

Now you have the foundation for answering the question "Why are you doing Atkins?" You're eating what your body is designed to absorb and utilize properly— the true and natural foods the earth provides. After that question, you may get some others—you'll be amazed at how much people have to say about Atkins. Let's take a look at some of the misinformation about the ANA you may be presented with:

Myth #1: *Lipolysis/ketosis is dangerous.*
Reality: Ketosis is not dangerous at all. Ketosis is the medical term for burning ketones, which are the byproduct of lipolysis, when you burn fat for energy. Your body has two built-in fuel delivery systems—one runs on glucose (also known as blood sugar), the other on fat. Because of the way we eat in our culture, the vast majority of people primarily use one of these systems— the glucose-burning one. When your body doesn't get sufficient carbohydrate in the foods you eat to burn for energy—you have only about two days' worth stored in your cells—it begins to burn fat, including body fat. This process of using fat instead of glucose to fuel your body is perfectly natural, safe and desirable. Burning fat instead of glucose to fuel your body is why you lose weight when you do Atkins. Ketosis occurs primarily in the weight-loss phases of the ANA, when carbohydrates are restricted most dramatically.

Even many doctors confuse ketosis with ketoacidosis, a life-threatening condition that affects insulin dependent diabetics. The two terms sound similar, but that's the only connection. Ketosis is simply a shorthand way to say your body is burning stored fat instead of glucose as its primary fuel.

Myth #2: *All that meat, butter and cheese will raise your cholesterol.*
Reality: Actually, just the opposite is true. Most people doing Atkins see a drop in the small dense LDL particles that cause plaque on the arteries and a rise in

their HDL cholesterol, the kind that is protective of your heart. And virtually everyone who does Atkins sees a dramatic drop in their triglycerides. On a low fat diet (which is necessarily a high carb diet), triglycerides (another type of blood fat) often go up and HDL goes down, which is just the opposite of what you want. In the last two years, research results comparing individuals following Atkins with those doing low fat programs have consistently confirmed what many doctors have observed in their practices: The risk factors for heart disease improve on Atkins. Some research has demonstrated that the combination of high triglycerides and low HDL—and not total cholesterol—may actually be the most important predictor of heart disease and stroke.

Myth #3: *Atkins can't be healthy, because you don't eat any fruits or vegetables.*
Reality: Wrong. On the ANA, you will get more nutrients from vegetables (and eventually, fruits) than you get in the typical American diet. People who have not read Dr. Atkins' books often mistakenly think the first phase of Atkins, known as Induction, is the whole plan. It is true that in the first phase you do not eat any fruit and limit vegetables to three cups daily, but Induction lasts a minimum of two weeks. Its purpose is to drastically reduce the amount of sugar entering your bloodstream and to jump-start your weight loss. What you are supposed to eat are nutrient-packed leafy greens such as broccoli, spinach or kale. In fact, you can satisfy the USDA's five-a-day guideline by eating the two

cups of salad greens, one cup of other vegetables such as broccoli and the half avocado that you are allowed on Induction.

As soon as you move to the Ongoing Weight Loss phase, you can add berries to your program. In the later phases of the ANA, you can eat more and more vegetables and fruit; the only restriction is that you concentrate on the plant foods that pack the most nutritious punch. By the time you are in Lifetime Maintenance, if you are like many people, you can eat virtually any plant food, although you will be advised to moderate the amount and frequency of the higher carb fruits and vegetables.

Myth #4: *You don't have to exercise to lose weight while doing Atkins.*
Reality: Wrong again. Exercise is integral to the ANA. It is the combination of controlled carbohydrate eating and regular physical activity that will keep you slim and at your healthiest best. It is not an optional part of the ANA; regular physical activity is mandatory for feeling good and for maximizing and maintaining weight loss. It also helps tone your body so that any flabbiness that might result from weight loss is minimized. (Even obese individuals can engage in low-impact programs such as chair exercises or water aerobics, after getting their doctor's go-ahead.)

During the first week of Induction, continue your usual exercise regimen. If you wish to increase your exercise level, you can do so the second week. For those of you who are not currently exercising, start thinking about what activities will work for you once you complete the first week of Induction. More information on establishing a fitness regimen can be found in Chapter 8.

Myth #5: *Eating large amounts of protein leaches calcium from your bones and interferes with calcium absorption.*
Reality: This is another myth that research has disproved. Your body will excrete a bit more calcium in the urine than usual when you are in Induction and losing excess water, but then your calcium balance returns to normal with no long-term effects. And recent research with older adults has shown that eating a high protein diet not only does not weaken your bones, it actually strengthens them if you also take a calcium supplement (as the Atkins program recommends).

Myth #6: *Eating all that protein is dangerous for your kidneys.*
Reality: This may be the biggest myth of all. There is absolutely no evidence for this common myth—not a single study shows that a high protein, low carbohydrate nutritional program damages normal kidneys. There are, however, studies showing that it can be problematic for an individual with kidney disease to consume too much animal protein. **If you have kidney disease, of course, you do have to sharply restrict your protein intake and shouldn't be doing Atkins without medical supervision.**

Myth #7: *The only reason Atkins works is because you eat fewer calories.*

Reality: While people may end up eating fewer calories while doing Atkins, this happens only because they're less hungry and no longer obsessed with food or craving carbohydrates. On Atkins, there is no restriction on calories. You can eat as much of the allowed foods as you need to feel satisfied. This, however, is not a license to gorge. If you restrict your carbs as instructed, you will lose weight.

> *I've found that my tastes really have changed on Atkins. My cravings have disappeared and sugary desserts usually taste too sweet to me now. Another thing that's changed is my attitude toward doubters. I used to avoid confrontation by telling people I was on a no-sugar diet. Now I arm myself with information and go tooth and nail with opponents! I love turning skeptics into participants. Almost as much as I loved having all my clothes taken in!*
>
> —Paul McDougal, lost 25 pounds

Myth #8: *The weight lost on Atkins is mostly water weight, not fat.*

Reality: On any weight-loss plan, during the first few days or even the first week, some of the weight lost will simply be water. Soon after, the body balances things out and restores the water you lose. When you follow a controlled carbohydrate eating plan, however, your body switches from burning carbohydrate to primarily burning stored fat—that would be the fat you see rolling over your waistband and bulging at your thighs. After the first week, you can be sure that the weight coming off is fat. All you need to do is watch the inches drop off your measurements and slide into those jeans that used to be too tight.

That ends our lesson in educating skeptics and should also have taken care of any doubts or questions that may have lingered in your own mind. If you have any others, more information of this kind can be found in Part Five, "Frequently Asked Questions." Now you're probably chomping at the bit to start doing Atkins. You're on your way!

We have one last task for you before you begin. So you won't forget (and though it's hard to believe, you may eventually forget these things), fill out our "Where I Am Today" sheet beginning on the opposite page. After you've finished filling in this information, Chapter 4 will explain exactly how the first phase of Atkins, called Induction, works.

▶ Food for Thought

Take a moment to answer these questions—you'll be glad you did. Not only will they help you better understand where you stand right now, looking back on your responses several weeks, and even months, from now will offer you a crystal-clear picture of the progress and positive changes you've made in your life. And that's a reward you won't want to miss.

"WHERE I AM TODAY"

Had you ever before considered the fact that our bodies were designed this way many eons ago and that they probably weren't meant to consume the kinds of foods Americans eat today? Have you ever gone an entire day without eating a single processed food?

_____

_____

_____

Test your knowledge. Jot down a list with everything you knew, thought you knew, or had heard about Atkins before you picked up this book. Next to each of these things, using the knowledge you have now, write _true_ or _false_. Where false, make a note explaining why it's false.

_____

_____

_____

Looking at your list, think about why people get stuck in a mindset or way of doing things and become so averse to change. What motivates naysayers? Do you consider yourself to have an open mind? Have you ever heard yourself say, "That's just the way it's done," or "We've always done it this way"?

_____

_____

_____

PART TWO

How to Do Atkins

4 ▶ The Big Picture

I used to drive a truck all day, eating fast food and snacking as I made deliveries. It's no wonder I weighed 450 pounds. A customer of mine told me about Atkins and gave me a copy of Dr. Atkins' New Diet Revolution *and some Atkins vitamins. She said, "Try Atkins for 14 days, and something will change in your life." I felt I owed it to her so I got started two days later. Surprisingly, I never craved carbs. Although I felt fatigued at first, I knew that was normal and a sign that my new way of eating was working. After a few weeks, I started to feel better than I had since high school, and after 11 months, I'd lost 195 pounds. I started to exercise and now I run and lift weights. I used to go watch my friends play softball. Last summer, I was asked to fill in for an absent player. No one had ever asked me before. I also started dating and now have a steady girlfriend. Losing weight has opened up my whole world, and it's a way of eating I can stick with for the rest of my life.*

—Donnie Moore, lost 195 pounds

Okay, now that you have a basic understanding of why Atkins works, it's time to get down to business. You're about to learn how to use this safe, incredibly effective approach to shed those extra pounds, once and for all! Let's get started. The Atkins Nutritional Approach™ (ANA) consists of four carefully designed phases: Induction, Ongoing Weight Loss (OWL), Pre-Maintenance and Lifetime Maintenance. It is very important that you follow the program through all four phases. If you view doing Atkins as a quick way to lose weight—instead of a major shift in the way you eat for life—you will almost certainly gain the weight back and all will be for naught. Remember, this is not a diet; this is a lifelong plan for achieving optimum health.

The first phase, **Induction**, is the crucial period during which you jump-start your weight loss by shifting your body's metabolism. By limiting your carbohydrate intake to 20 grams of Net Carbs daily, mostly in the form of vegetables, your body will exhaust its stored supply of carbohydrate within the first 48 hours and gradually make the switch to primarily burning stored fat for energy. The Induction phase must last a minimum of two weeks, but if you have a lot of weight to lose, you can safely stay on it for many months if you choose.

During the first two weeks, you eat fish, poultry, eggs, beef, tofu and other foods high in protein. You will also eat three cups of salad greens (with low carb dressing) or two cups of salad and one cup of low carb vegetables, such as broccoli, zucchini or any of the veggies from a long list of others you will find begining on page 78. You're also allowed up to four ounces of cheese (one ounce is about the size of an individually wrapped American cheese slice or one-inch cube) and half of a small avocado each day. After two weeks on Induction, you can also add an ounce of nuts or seeds, which is roughly a small handful (see "Nibble on Nuts" on pages 150–151), to your daily intake so long as they don't interfere with weight loss. (All of this will be spelled out for you in the "Acceptable Induction Foods" list in the next chapter.)

While on Induction—and beyond—it is important that you take two daily nutritional supplements: a multivitamin/mineral and essential fatty acids (EFA). In fact, a key component of doing Atkins is supplementing your meals with vitamins, minerals and essential fatty acids. (Atkins Nutritionals has specially formulated supplements to support the nutritional needs of those following a controlled carbohydrate lifestyle. They are available in natural foods stores and on *www.atkins.com.*) So is establishing an exercise routine (see Chapter 8). Doing Atkins is like sitting on a three-legged stool. You need to follow a controlled carbohydrate dietary approach, exercise regularly and take vitamin and mineral supplements to ensure all your nutritional needs are being met. Although you will be eating a whole foods diet, you cannot be assured that you are getting all the nutrients you need from food. Anyone who has been eating the typical American diet is likely to be deficient in nutrients because the soil in which our food grows is often depleted. Moreover, we need additional nutritional support because our bodies are under constant stress from environmental toxins.

The second phase of the ANA is called **Ongoing Weight Loss**, OWL for short. During this phase, you continue to eat high-quality proteins and fats, along with your salad greens and other acceptable vegetables. But week by week, you will add back nutrient-rich carbohydrates such as more vegetables, fresh cheese, nuts, seeds, berries and perhaps other low glycemic fruits like plums and grapefruit, and legumes, depending on how they affect your weight loss. You do this by bumping up your daily Net Carb count by 5 grams each week until your weight loss stops for more than a week. At that point, you'll back down by 5 grams and you should have discovered your own personal carbohydrate threshold—the number of daily grams of Net Carbs you can consume while still losing weight. For most people, that number is somewhere between 40 and 60 grams of Net Carbs per day. We call that your Critical Carbohydrate Level for Losing, or CCLL for short. You'll stay on OWL until you are within 5 or 10 pounds of your goal weight.

Pre-Maintenance is the third phase of the ANA and it is just what it sounds like—this is your final "practice" period for adopting this new way of eating that will keep you healthy and slim for the rest of your life. The point of Pre-Maintenance is to slow your weight loss down to an almost imperceptible rate so that your new eating habits become fully ingrained. Each week, you'll add another 10 daily grams of Net Carbs—or treat yourself to an extra 20 to 30 grams of nutrient-dense foods twice a week—as long as you continue to gradually lose (less than a pound a week). If your weight loss stops completely, cut back by 5 or 10 grams until it resumes. This is your revised carbohydrate threshold, the number of daily grams of Net Carbs you will consume until you reach your goal weight.

The final phase of the ANA is called **Lifetime Maintenance**. Again, its name defines it. This is your permanent way of eating, which will enable you to maintain your goal weight for the rest of your life. When you reach this phase, you can begin to enjoy an even wider variety of foods. You'll always, of course, skip the white "junk" food, but now you can spread your carb allowance over a broad selection of whole grains, vegetables and fruit. Most people can maintain their weight by consuming somewhere between 45 and 100 grams of Net Carbs per day. Someone who exercises an hour or more each day or has a job with physical demands may be able to consume an even higher amount. This magic number is your Atkins Carbohydrate Equilibrium (ACE), the number of grams of Net Carbs you can consume without gaining or losing weight. Being male or young gives you an advantage; older people, including women in menopause, tend to have a lower ACE. To a certain extent, your genes also play a role.

That's the ANA, in a nutshell. Sounds eminently doable, doesn't it? Now that you've got the big picture, the rest of Part Two and Part Three of this book will be devoted to taking you, step by step, through your first two weeks of Induction. We'll talk again about the subsequent phases of the ANA in Part Four, just before we leave you poised for a swift and enjoyable flight to the thinner, stronger, more energetic you.

➤ The 20 Rules of Induction

As previously mentioned, Induction can last 14 days, or you can safely continue it for months. While this first two-week phase of the ANA should not be confused with the complete Atkins program, doing it exactly as you're instructed is critical. Try your own version of it or "cheat" here and there, and you are in danger of missing the boat: You won't lose weight the way you ought to, you may not feel well, you may conclude that Atkins doesn't work, and you just might abandon the opportunity of a lifetime. So perhaps we should rethink this: Consider the first two weeks doing Atkins to be a time of complete commitment, during which you give yourself over to your new way of eating with your heart and soul.

Are you ready? Here are the rules. Memorize them as though your life depended on it:

1. **Do not skip meals.** Eat three regular-size meals a day or four or five smaller meals.
2. **Do not go more than six waking hours without eating.** Some people may need a snack at the four-hour mark.
3. **Eat enough protein.** Consume it in the form of poultry, fish, shellfish, meat and eggs, and eat enough to feel comfortably full but not stuffed.

4. **Eat liberal amounts of pure, natural fats.**
   These include: olive oil; butter; mayonnaise;
   cream; seed, nut or vegetable oils (preferably
   expeller- or cold-pressed) such as sesame, safflower, walnut, flaxseed, peanut, canola, and
   corn oil. You can also eat tub margarine-type
   spreads that are free of trans fats (hydrogenated oil), which are available in natural
   foods stores and some supermarkets. Natural
   fats are also in protein foods such as meat,
   fish, poultry, eggs and cheese.

5. **Avoid all types of hydrogenated oils completely.** These are found in shortening and most
   margarines. They are also in most packaged
   baked goods, but you will not be eating these
   high carb foods in Induction and, in fact, should
   eliminate them from your diet permanently.

6. **Eat no more than 20 grams a day of Net
   Carbs.** Most of the 20 grams must come from
   salad greens and other vegetables. (You may eat
   approximately three cups—loosely packed—of
   leafy greens and other salad vegetables or two
   cups of salad plus one cup of other vegetables
   (see Chapter 5). You may also have one or
   two portions of certain low carb products so
   long as you stay at or below 20 grams of Net
   Carbs.

7. **Eat absolutely no fruit, regular bread, pasta,
   grains, starchy vegetables, legumes or anything made with flour or sugar in the initial
   phases of weight loss.**

8. **Eat no dairy products other than cheese, cream or butter.**

9. **Do not eat nuts or seeds in the first two weeks.** (If you stay on Induction, you may add one ounce of nuts and/or seeds in week three. Peanut butter and other nut spreads should not be hydrogenated. You will recognize nonhydrogenated nut butters because the oil sits on the top of the contents and has to be stirred before use.)

10. **Eat only the foods you find on "The Master List"** (see Chapter 5).

11. **Let your appetite be your guide.** Eat whenever you're hungry, but stop as soon as you are pleasantly full.

12. **Have a small, low carb snack if you are hungry between meals.**

13. **If you're not hungry at mealtimes, eat a small, low carb snack with your nutritional supplements.**

14. **Don't assume any food is low in carbohydrate.** Check the carb count on every package or use a carbohydrate gram counter.

15. **When you eat out, watch for hidden carbs.** Flour, cornstarch and sugar are often ingredients in gravies, sauces and dressings.

16. **Count each packet of artificial sweetener as 1 gram of Net Carbs.** Use sucralose (Splenda®), saccharin (Sweet 'N Low®) or acesulfame-K (Sweet One®) to sweeten things.

17. **Avoid caffeine in the form of coffee, tea and soft drinks.** Excessive caffeine can cause unstable blood sugar and make you crave sugar.

18. **Drink at least eight 8-ounce glasses of water each day.**

19. **If you are constipated, mix a tablespoon or more of psyllium husks in a cup or more of water and drink daily.** Or mix ground flaxseed into a shake or sprinkle unprocessed wheat bran flakes on a salad or vegetables. Fiber need not be counted in your daily carb count.

20. **Take a good-quality daily multivitamin— one that includes the minerals potassium, magnesium and calcium—as well as an essential fatty acids supplement.** Unless you are iron deficient, your multivitamin should not include iron.

► Food for Thought

Once again, these questions are designed to help you track your progress. If you don't know your accurate weight, now is the time to step on the scale and record it. Measurements and health indicators will come in handy as another way to gauge your results, as well as inspire you to keep pushing toward your goals. If you're unpleasantly surprised by some of the numbers you record, relax; by deciding to do Atkins, you've already taken the most important step on the road to achieving better health and a slimmer body.

What is your . . .

Present weight: _____

Goal weight: _____

Present clothing size: _____

Goal clothing size: _____

Chest: _____

Waist: _____

Hips: _____

Upper arms: _____

Thighs: _____

Total cholesterol: _____

LDL cholesterol: _____

HDL cholesterol: _____

Triglycerides: _____

Blood pressure: _____

Glucose (blood sugar): _____

When you look back over the past week . . .

How much exercise did you get?

_____
_____
_____

How has your mood been?

_____
_____
_____

How has your energy level been?

_____
_____
_____

How well have you been sleeping?

_____
_____
_____

Have you been craving sugar or other carbs?

_____
_____
_____

5 ► The Master List

You've read the rules. Now for the ingredients you'll need to employ them. Get to know the "Acceptable Induction Foods" list, which is made up of the sumptuous foods you'll be eating exclusively for at least the next two weeks. You may have to read it several times—it includes plenty of foods you've been instructed not to eat in the past when you've tried to shed pounds the low fat way. But don't call your eye doctor; the foods you see listed *really* will help you lose weight and keep it off . . . permanently.

While we know that it is not always possible, we strongly recommend that you eat organic vegetables (and fruit in later phases of Atkins), which have not been treated with pesticides and artificial fertilizers. Likewise, look for meats and poultry that have not been treated with hormones, antibiotics or nitrates.

► **Acceptable Induction Foods**

FOODS YOU DO <u>NOT</u> NEED TO LIMIT

- Poultry
- Fish
- Shellfish
- Meat
- Eggs

Exceptions:
- Oysters and mussels are higher in carbs than other shellfish, so eat no more than four ounces a day.
- Processed meats, such as ham, bacon, pepperoni, salami, hot dogs and other luncheon meats—and some fish—may be cured with sugar or contain fillers that contribute carbs.
- Avoid meat and fish products cured with nitrates, which are known carcinogens.
- Also beware of products that are not exclusively meat, fish or fowl, such as imitation crabmeat, fish sticks, meatloaf and all breaded foods.
- Do not consume more than four ounces of organ meats a day.

FOODS YOU <u>DO</u> NEED TO LIMIT

Cheese: 3 to 4 ounces per day

All cheeses contain some carbohydrate. You can consume three to four ounces daily of full-fat, firm, soft and semi-soft aged cheeses (for example, cheddar, Swiss, Gouda, goat cheese, mozzarella, blue cheese). Count one ounce of cheese as 1 gram of Net Carbs. Full-fat cream cheese also is permitted, as are cheeses made from soy or rice, but check the carbohydrate content so that you consume no more than 4 grams of Net Carbs from cheese.

Not Allowed:
- Cottage cheese
- Farmer cheese
- Ricotta cheese
- Other fresh cheeses (not aged)
- Reduced fat or low calorie cheeses
- Processed cheeses such as cheese spreads

Other Dairy

- Butter (unlimited)
- 2 to 4 ounces (4 tablespoons to half a cup) of light or heavy cream **OR** sour cream

Salad Vegetables: 2 to 3 cups per day

You can have two to three loosely packed cups per day of the following raw vegetables:

- Alfalfa sprouts
- Arugula
- Cabbage
- Celery
- Chicory
- Chives
- Cucumber
- Daikon
- Endive
- Escarole
- Fennel
- Jicama
- Lettuce (all types)
- Mâche
- Mushrooms
- Parsley
- Peppers
- Radicchio
- Radishes
- Romaine
- Scallions
- Sorrel
- Spinach
- Tomato
- Watercress

Or any other leafy green vegetables.

Cooked Vegetables: 1 cup per day

You can have one cup (measured cooked) per day of these vegetables if salad does not exceed two cups. A few vegetables, such as spinach or tomatoes, that cook down significantly, should be measured raw. Some of the following vegetables are slightly higher in carbohydrate content than the salad vegetables:

- Artichoke
- Artichoke hearts
- Asparagus
- Bamboo shoots
- Bean sprouts
- Beet greens
- Bok choy
- Broccoli
- Broccoli rabe
- Brussels sprouts
- Cabbage
- Cauliflower
- Celery root
- Chard
- Collard greens
- Dandelion greens
- Eggplant
- Hearts of palm
- Kale
- Kohlrabi
- Leeks
- Okra

- Pumpkin
- Rhubarb
- Sauerkraut
- Snow peas
- Spaghetti squash
- String or wax beans
- Summer squash
- Tomato
- Turnips
- Water chestnuts
- Zucchini or summer squash

Note that certain vegetables appear on both lists.

Garnishes

- Crumbled crisp bacon (look for nitrate-free products)
- Grated cheese (figure into your cheese count)
- Minced hard-boiled egg
- Sautéed mushrooms (figure into your vegetable count)
- Spices and herbs (as long as they contain no added sugar)
- Sliced or chopped onion

Salad Dressings

- Oil and vinegar
- Salad dressings made without sugar or corn syrup (should be no more than 2 grams of Net Carbs per serving)

Not Allowed:
- Balsamic vinegar (contains added sugar)
- Rice vinegar made with added sugar
- Salad dressings made with added sugar or corn syrup

Condiments

- Caponata (eggplant relish)
- Mayonnaise (regular, not low fat)
- Mustard (not honey mustard)
- Horseradish
- Pesto (after first two weeks of Induction)
- Pickles (but not "bread and butter" or other sweet pickles)
- Soy sauce (tamari, others made without wheat)
- Tabasco® sauce
- Tapanade (black olive puree)
- Worcestershire sauce

Also, low carb sauces such as ketchup, hoisin, and sweet and sour made without added sugar are acceptable. Always check carb counts. A serving should contain no more than 2 grams of Net Carbs.

Not Allowed:
- Barbecue sauce
- Ketchup made with added sugar
- Pickle relish
- Russian dressing
- Cranberry sauce

Also unacceptable is any sauce with added sugar, corn syrup or flour, such as steak sauce, packaged gravies, etc.

Oils

You may use any type of oil, preferably cold-pressed or expeller-pressed. Olive oil or butter is preferred but you may use margarine-like spreads made of vegetable oils as long as they contain no trans fats (hydrogenated oil).

Artificial Sweeteners

The words *sugarless*, *sugar-free* or *no sugar added* are not sufficient. Look at carbohydrate counts. We recommend the following sweeteners:

- Sucralose (marketed as Splenda®)
- Saccharin (marketed as Sweet 'N Low®)
- Acesulfame-K (Sweet One®)

Note: Most chewing gum, breath mints, cough syrups and cough drops are filled with sugar or other caloric sweeteners and must be avoided. However, sugar-free products are available.

Beverages

Be sure to drink a minimum of eight 8-ounce glasses of water each day, including:

- Filtered water
- Mineral water
- Spring water
- Tap water

The following beverages are acceptable, but should be consumed only in addition to the 64 ounces of water:

- Decaffeinated coffee or tea
- Diet soda made with one of the acceptable artificial sweeteners (no more than three a day; be sure to count the carbs)
- Essence-flavored seltzer (must say "no calories")
- Herb tea (without barley or any fruit sugar added)
- Clear broth/bouillon (not all brands; read the label)
- Club soda

Not Allowed:
- Coffee substitutes made from grains
- Alcoholic beverages
- Caffeinated cola drinks
- Fruit or vegetable juices

Special Category Foods

Each day you can also eat the following:

- 10 to 20 olives
- Half a small avocado

- 2 to 3 tablespoons of lemon juice or lime juice (count 3 grams of Net Carbs for 2 tablespoons)
- If you stay on Induction past week two, you can add one ounce of nuts and/or seeds to your daily intake.

Note: These foods occasionally slow down weight loss in some people, and may need to be avoided at first. If you seem to be losing slowly, moderate your intake of these foods or avoid them altogether.

ATKINS LOW CARB INGREDIENTS

These ingredients can come in handy when planning meals:

- Atkins™ Sugar Free Syrups
- Atkins™ Sweet Dressings
- Atkins Quick Quisine™ Sugar Free Pancake Syrup
- Atkins Quick Quisine™ Ketch-a-Tomato Sauce
- Atkins Quick Quisine™ Barbecue Sauce
- Atkins Quick Quisine™ Steak Sauce
- Atkins Quick Quisine™ Teriyaki Sauce
- Atkins Quick Quisine™ Bake Mix
- Atkins Kitchen™ Quick & Easy Bread Mix
- Atkins Quick Quisine™ Pancake & Waffle Mixes
- Atkins Quick Quisine™ Bake Mixes

ATKINS LOW CARB CONVENIENCE FOODS

It is important that you eat primarily unprocessed foods, but some controlled carb food products can come in handy when you are unable to find appropriate foods, can't take time for a meal or need a quick snack. Atkins products suitable for Induction include:

- Atkins Advantage™ Bars
- Atkins Advantage™ Shakes (as mixes or in ready-to-drink cans)
- Atkins Morning Start™ Breakfast Bars
- Atkins Bakery™ Ready-to-Eat Sliced Bread (one slice)

Note: Do not consume more than two servings of low carb alternative foods during Induction, and remember that you still must count your grams of Net Carbs. If you have trouble losing weight you may want to replace these products with protein and fat whole foods during the Induction phase.

➤ Food for Thought

You know you are going to have to eat, so don't let meals take you by surprise. A little preparation can help you avoid pitfalls and achieve success more efficiently. Be sure that you have everything at your fingertips—and in your fridge—to do Atkins right by asking yourself the following questions.

Have you removed (or placed off-limits) foods that contain sugar and white flour, and other processed foods (junk foods)?

_____

_____

_____

If not, what do you need to do to ensure that you are not tempted by these foods?

_____

_____

_____

Have you stocked your refrigerator, freezer and pantry with appropriate low carb foods?

_____

_____

_____

If not, what do you still have to buy?

_____

_____

_____

Have you thought about the meals you will be making your first few days doing Atkins?

_____

_____

_____

What Atkins-appropriate snacks do you have on hand?

_____

_____

_____

If you will be eating out, have you thought about how you will navigate the menu?

_____

_____

_____

6 ► Your First Week on Atkins

I started Induction on a Saturday. I have to admit that I felt terrible for the first 36 hours, but I woke up Tuesday morning feeling like a whole new person. I literally leapt out of bed. The cravings during the first week were tough, but I followed the book to a tee. It said, "If you're hungry, eat." So that's what I did. I've never had more energy or felt more high on life. I realize now that this is what it's like to feel normal.

—Bob Keown, lost 63 pounds

As you embark on the first few days of your new lifestyle, you are probably filled with excitement and expectations. That is as it should be. You are making a major commitment toward your dream of improving your health, your energy, your sense of well-being and your looks.

Time for a reality check: The first week on Atkins may not be, punning aside, a piece of cake. Almost everyone who has completed the Induction phase will tell you these first days can be the hardest. Just like quitting smoking or giving up any addiction, going cold turkey on sugar (and often caffeine at the same time) can be a tough transition. But after reading this book, we hope you'll understand that kicking the carb habit is vitally important to your long-term health and well-being. Remember, you are making a wise choice that will enable you to live a healthier life.

▶ Before Your Body Makes the Shift

Remember that your body has two main fuel sources: fat and carbohydrate. Your objective in the first few days of doing Atkins is to switch your body from burning carbohydrate (in the form of blood sugar) for energy to primarily burning fat, including body fat. That is how you will lose weight by doing Atkins. So let's walk through what's likely to happen as you start your new lifestyle and your body shifts its way of producing energy. Understand that everyone has a different metabolism, meaning you will lose weight at your own individual pace. That said, in the first few days, most people share the following two experiences:

1. **You won't lose weight immediately.** During the first few days of Induction, the scale may not budge. But shortly afterward, you'll likely see a big drop, which is due largely to the initial loss of excess water weight. This happens at the beginning of any weight-loss program, but the effect can be more dra-

matic on Atkins, because the body burns off its stores of carbohydrate in the first few days—and a lot of retained water goes with it. Plus you are taking in fewer foods with high water content. (There are four molecules of water attached to every molecule of carbohydrate.)

2. **You'll crave carbohydrates.** While you're depleting your body's stores of carbohydrate and before you've begun to burn fat, you may still have to battle cravings for bagels, cookies, chips and other high carb foods for a few days. Be assured that this will not last! Stay focused, and before you know it, you'll be coming out on the other side with no cravings and feeling fantastic.

▶ **Possible First-Week Symptoms**

My first two days on Atkins were absolutely awful. I've never smoked, drank or taken drugs, so I was completely unprepared for what withdrawal feels like. I had the shakes and felt so bad that I almost stopped. I kept thinking, "No, I can't do this!" but I pressed on and got through it. By the end of the second day, I felt fine. In fact, I was sleeping better at night and feeling more energetic during the day. I had so much energy that I started walking three miles every day.

—Evelyn Velasquez, lost 51 pounds

Just about everyone experiences a few days in which they struggle with food cravings, but the range of other symptoms is highly personal. Some people experience few or no other symptoms; others have an array of reactions. It is unlikely that you will experience all of the following symptoms, but we do want you to understand what could occur and what you can do to alleviate them in case they do happen to you. The most important thing to remember is that these symptoms are perfectly normal and they are only temporary. Everyone's body reacts to changes differently. Depending upon what you have been eating until now, you may or may not actually experience withdrawal from carbs.

Symptom: *Carb withdrawal as exhibited by fatigue, light-headedness, headache, irritability or cold sweats.*

Cause: Some people experience these classic withdrawal symptoms as a result of suddenly being deprived of a food to which they were, knowingly or unknowingly, addicted. Many people have addictions to foods they consume every day without being aware of them. You may have one or more of these symptoms. Common offenders are caffeine, sugar, wheat and other foods capable of quickly changing blood sugar levels. If you are going to experience carbohydrate withdrawal, the symptoms can begin by the end of the first day on Atkins. At worst they can last up to five days. In most people they are manageable and are usually gone by the third day.

How to deal with it: *Option 1*) Go cold turkey and hang in there. Bad as they seem, experiencing withdrawal symptoms is really good news. The withdrawal process is usually completed within three days, and afterward you should feel better than ever.

Option 2) If you cannot stay the course and power through withdrawal, wean yourself off your addiction(s) gradually by first removing sugar and refined flour from your diet for four days, and then return to Induction. The more severe your withdrawal symptoms, the more you stand to gain from abandoning the food(s) that causes them.

If you continue to experience these symptoms, slow down the weight-loss process until your body adapts by adding another helping of vegetables to your meals each day; alternatively, add one or two ounces of nuts or seeds, which add some more carbs. Full of healthy fats, they make a perfect between-meal snack and are more convenient than veggies to eat on the run. Salted nuts also can add sodium, which slows down water loss—and with it mineral depletion. Although your body will likely adjust during the second week, there's no good reason to feel weak and sickly for even one day. After the symptoms abate, return to the lower level of carb intake.

Symptom: *Fatigue, weakness or light-headedness, and ascent weakness (sudden weakness or heaviness in the legs on an incline or climbing stairs).* A small percentage of people experience such symptoms at the

end of the first week of Induction following the initial
diuretic effect. (By this time, weakness will no longer
indicate carb withdrawal.)

Cause: One or more of these symptoms usually
means that weight loss is occurring too fast for your
particular metabolism. Losing water weight rapidly
can deplete you of such minerals, also known as electrolytes, as calcium, magnesium and potassium. These
play an important role in keeping your body in balance. Sweating as a result of hot weather and/or vigorous exercise can aggravate these symptoms.

How to deal with it: If you are doing Atkins properly, you are drinking a minimum of eight glasses of
water a day and taking your nutritional supplements,
both of which will minimize the likelihood of these
symptoms. If you are exercising a lot or the weather
is hot, you may need more fluid. Your multivita-
min/mineral should be full of minerals. If you have
not been taking a supplement, begin to do so immediately. To restore lost minerals, you can also consume
salty broth or potassium-rich foods such as parsley,
avocado, spinach, broccoli, almonds or sunflower
seeds. Also be sure you are eating three full meals or
four or five smaller meals. Remember not to skip
meals, even if you're not hungry, and to have snacks
if you get hungry between meals. If weight loss is
still too rapid, move beyond the 20 grams of Net
Carbs per day by adding more salad or vegetables.

BETWEEN-MEAL NIBBLING

Snacking can be your secret weapon for weight control, so long as you select nutritious low carb foods.

Americans love snack foods so much that on average they get about 25 percent of their daily calories from junk food such as potato chips. High in calories and empty carbs, they are practically devoid of nutrition. Sweet snacks are just as popular. According to the Snack Food Association, sales of snacks of all sorts now top $30 billion a year. Is it any wonder that well over half of all American adults are now overweight, as are nearly a third of all kids?

Conventional snack foods are made from inexpensive, highly refined ingredients such as white flour, cornmeal, corn syrup and white sugar. Even worse, they're high in trans fats (also known as hydrogenated or partially hydrogenated vegetable oils), a dangerous substance that is a major culprit behind clogged arteries. Here are some strategies for fighting back:

- **Know your enemy.** If you're aware of how bad these foods are for you, you're better able to resist them. "Bad" carb foods are also full of dangerous trans fats, artificial flavorings and preservatives. Read the ingredients label—it's enough to make you never touch the stuff.

- **Purge your pantry.** If junk foods aren't there, you can't eat them. Your kids might complain, but junk food is no better for them than it is for you—and if you set the example, they'll find it easier to follow.
- **Avoid certain aisles.** Most of the snack foods are concentrated in the very supermarket aisles an Atkins follower should not be in. Also stay away from the food displays at the checkout by choosing the "no snack" counter if there is one.

Doing Atkins doesn't mean not eating between meals. On the contrary, snacking can help you avoid getting so hungry that you pig out at your next meal. There's no shortage of enjoyable and convenient low carb choices. String cheese sticks or single-portion cheese rounds are handy and delicious. Olives are full of healthy fats. An Atkins Advantage™ Bar can satisfy a sweet tooth. For a convenient and satisfying hot snack, try low carb instant soup. A piece of chicken or a slice of roast beef and other meat snacks are good choices, but read the labels carefully to avoid added carbs.

If crunch is what you crave, try celery sticks stuffed with cream cheese. Once you are past the first two weeks of Induction, you can also enjoy a handful of seeds or nuts or peanut butter on your celery sticks. (See "Nibble on Nuts" beginning on page 150.)

If you crave chocolate (and who doesn't?), another option is an Atkins Advantage™ Ready-to-Drink Chocolate Shake or Chocolate Peanut Butter Bar.

In the second phase of Atkins, known as Ongoing Weight Loss, you can also enjoy berries with cream as a snack choice. As your carb intake increases, typically by Pre-Maintenance, you can also snack on grapefruit, kiwis, cherries, apples and melons, preferably with some nuts or cheese. For a fun snack on a hot day, have some frozen grapes or ice pops made with artificially sweetened homemade lemonade.

Symptom: *Leg cramps.* During the first week on Induction, some people experience leg cramps, which often occur at night.

Cause: Leg cramps are another result of electrolyte loss due to dehydration.

How to deal with it: If you're taking your multivitamin/mineral and leg cramps still bother you, you may want to add a multimineral supplement or take extra calcium along with stepping up your intake of water.

Note: If you continue to feel bad after several days, you may want to see your physician to determine whether your symptoms indicate that you have the flu or another condition unrelated to doing Atkins.

Symptom: *Constipation.* Irregularity is also common in the first week of the Atkins Nutritional Approach™ (ANA).

Cause: Any sudden dietary change can produce this result, as you may have noticed when you tried another weight-loss program or traveled in a different country.

How to deal with it: You may recall that rule number 19 of Induction is to use a fiber supplement for constipation. Your options include psyllium husks, ground flaxseed and unprocessed wheat or oat bran—all of which can be found in a health food store. Drink plenty of fluids, exercise and gradually increase the amount of fiber you use until constipation abates.

COPING WITH CONSTIPATION

When you begin Induction, you're probably making a big change in your eating habits. Your body needs a little time to adjust, and until it does, you may be constipated. Irregularity happens when you have fewer bowel movements than are normal for you, or when your stool is hard, dry and difficult to pass. Other symptoms of constipation include cramps, bloating, dull headache, backache and sluggishness.

Irregularity can happen for a wide variety of reasons. As a general rule, however, there are three main culprits:

1. Not eating enough dietary fiber
2. Not drinking enough water
3. Not getting enough exercise

The Fiber Factor

Put simply, dietary fiber is the indigestible part of plant foods. Fiber absorbs water and provides bulk to your stool, making it soft. Most vegetables are an excellent source of dietary fiber, and during Induction you'll be eating three cups a day. If you're experiencing constipation, however, you might be skimping on your portions.

Next, are you getting enough variety in your vegetables? Even if you're eating the full three cups, you might be shortchanging yourself fiberwise. Salad greens such as iceberg and romaine lettuce, for instance, are relatively low in fiber. Instead, use several different kinds of lettuce and other leafy greens such as watercress, arugula and spinach in your salad, along with other crisp raw vegetables, such as green bell pepper or celery. The fiber count per cup will go up considerably.

Choose carefully among the other vegetables on the permitted list. Broccoli, cauliflower, asparagus, string beans, snow peas and cabbage are particularly rich in fiber.

Drink Up!

To prevent constipation it is also essential to drink at least 64 ounces of water every day. You may

well be skimping in this department as well. Induction cuts out fruit juices, milk and soda pop.
You may also be cutting out or down on caffeinated beverages such as coffee, tea and colas.
That leaves you with a relatively limited choice of
drinks beyond plain water. Without realizing it,
you may not be drinking enough.

Make a conscious effort to drink more water
and mineral water and also switch to decaffeinated tea and coffee and try some of the many
interesting caffeine-free herbal teas—you'll find a
wide variety available. You can also add beef or
chicken broth. A cup about half an hour before
mealtime has the added advantage of cutting your
appetite.

Get Moving!

Fiber and fluid are very helpful for preventing and
relieving constipation, but they'll work a lot better
in tandem with exercise. Interestingly, although
doctors know this works, they don't know exactly
why. It could be that exercise helps move food
through your digestive tract a bit faster. It also
helps tone the abdominal muscles used in elimination. Whether or not you're constipated, daily exercise is an essential part of doing Atkins, so
now's a good time to start incorporating it into
your lifestyle!

Extra Help

If adding more fiber in the form of vegetables isn't doing the trick, try a dose of crushed flaxseed to relieve your constipation. This excellent natural remedy is available at any health food store. Stir two teaspoons into a glass of water and drink it down in the evening—you'll probably get results the next morning. You can also sprinkle it on a salad or stir it into a protein drink. Oat or unprocessed wheat bran flakes are other natural approaches. An alternative is a bulk-forming, sugar-free fiber supplement made from psyllium (Fiberall®, Metamucil®). These products are available as powders, capsules and wafers; use as directed on the package. Unless your doctor recommends them, don't use chemical or herbal laxatives or stool softeners. These products can cause uncomfortable cramping and diarrhea, and their effects may remain with you for several days.

► Fat Burning Begins

TURNAROUND TIME

At some point around day three, often quite suddenly, you'll begin to feel the benefits of burning fat and having a more stable blood sugar level. Some people may take as long as a week to feel this way. But then the inevitable breakthrough occurs. No more obsessing about food, hunger pangs vanish, your energy soars, your digestion improves, heartburn disappears and even your sleep is better. Many people say they have as much verve and vigor as they had in high school. Others report feeling simultaneously more alert and calm. Some experience a period of euphoria. Others say it's the first time in as long as they can remember that they feel, simply, normal.

> *You have to really commit to the first two weeks. During the first week of Induction, I felt faint and awful. But after 14 days, I felt like a new person. I had dropped 12 pounds and I was bursting with energy.*
>
> —*Luann Lockhart, lost 75 pounds*

FIND YOUR OWN WEIGHT-LOSS PACE

Although each individual is different, weight loss of four to eight pounds is typical in the first two weeks of Induction if the program is followed to the letter. Some people lose even more, others less. Men typically lose between four to eight pounds, women between three and six. People who are significantly overweight may lose weight faster than those with more modest weight goals. But understand that there is no magic number. You may be a fast loser or a maddeningly slow loser. But rest assured that after the first four or five days, you've lost all the water pounds you're going to lose.

From now on, every ounce—and every inch—that comes off is solely fat!

DON'T OBSESS ABOUT THE SCALE

Of course your objective is to slim down, but weighing yourself several times a day or even once a day is not going to make any difference. Because your weight normally fluctuates throughout the day and even from day to day, getting on the scale every other morning or even just twice a week is better than every day. Many people avoid the scale completely for the first two weeks so they can have a wonderful surprise waiting for them on Day 14. (You will have gotten some hints from the way your clothes are beginning to fit!)

WHAT IF YOU ARE NOT LOSING?

If you do get on the scale and notice that you are not losing by your fourth or fifth day, measure yourself to check if inches are coming off. If inches also are not disappearing, you need to get moving and exercise more. You should also make sure that you are consuming plenty of natural fat and not overconsuming protein. Eating more fat combined with eating fewer carbs stimulates your body to use fat instead of glucose (blood sugar) for energy. Protein is crucial for feeding your body, but if you eat huge amounts of protein it can actually get in the way of fat burning and stall weight loss. Eat until you are comfortably full but not stuffed. While you can consume more calories on Atkins and lose more weight than on a low fat program, it is possible to overconsume calories. It is also possible to eat too little and slow down your metabolism, and that is why it is important to eat at least three meals daily.

So, don't gorge on protein, and make sure you're getting plenty of the good fats, such as olive oil, oily fish (if you are someone who simply cannot eat fish, consider taking fish oil in capsules), butter and full-fat cheese along with the naturally occurring fats in your protein choices. These small adjustments should get you burning off the pounds.

Many people who have tried and failed to lose weight on a low fat program before turning to Atkins have a hard time believing that it is okay to eat fat. They think they can go Atkins one better by doing their own low fat version of the program. The truth is that it is not just okay to eat fat, providing it is natural fats and not hydrogenated oils, it is downright essential to eat fat to help jump-start fat burning.

STILL NOT LOSING?

Don't despair. Turn to page 111, where we discuss a condition called *metabolic resistance* and how to break through it.

I tell people that you have to be really rigorous on Induction because if you cheat in the first two weeks, you're setting yourself up to fail. If you binge on carbs, you're going to crave more carbs, which can make it really hard to get back on track. But once you "get it," it's incredibly easy to eat like this forever.

—Kerry Feather, lost 60 pounds

WATER WAYS

What you already know: You need to drink eight 8-ounce glasses of water every day.

What you don't know: Why?
Here are the reasons to fill up your cup:

- Believe it or not, without those magic eight, you could be walking around in a state of mild dehydration. That can result in fatigue and, more important when you're trying to lose weight, a slowed metabolism.
- Water is a significant component of bodily fluids, like digestive juices, blood and perspiration.
- It regulates body temperature and carries nutrients throughout the body.
- It is vital to all organ function and cell processes.
- Water is essential for digestion and elimination. Drinking plenty of water can also help prevent constipation. (See page 96.)
- It assists in maintaining the PH balance in the body.

VISUALIZING PORTION SIZES

The beginning of your weight-loss program is a good time to get a sense of what typical portion sizes translate to. This way, you can be in control of your portions and stay on plan.

Vegetables

Portion:	Think of:
1 cup green salad	A fist
½ cup cooked vegetables	A scoop of ice cream

Protein and Cheese

Portion:	Think of:
6 ounces beef, chicken or pork	Two decks of playing cards
1 ounce of cheese	A pair of dice
1 ounce of nuts	Two Ping-Pong balls or a small child's handful

Measurements

Portion:	Think of:
1 tablespoon	A tea bag
1 teaspoon	A thimble
1 cup	A fist or a baseball
¼ cup	A large egg

TIME FOR CONGRATULATIONS!

Whether it was easy or hard, whether you lost two pounds or eight pounds, you made it through your first week. So take a moment to pat yourself on the back. You've taken action and put your plan in motion. The hardest part is behind you, and what you have to look forward to is all good. Stay focused, stick to your plan and you will continue to feel better and start looking better, all while controlling carbs gets easier and easier.

In Chapter 7, we'll take you through your second week on the ANA and have a look at where you stand on Day 14.

► Food for Thought

It's time to take stock again and document where you are after just one week on the ANA. Fill out your vital statistics and answer the questions below on Day 7 of Induction. You'll do this again on Day 14 and can compare your numbers and answers.

"DAY 7: WHERE I AM TODAY"

Date you started doing Atkins: _____

Present weight: _____

Pounds lost: _____

Goal weight: _____

Present clothing size: _____

Goal clothing size: _____

Present chest: _____

Inches lost: _____

Present waist: _____

Inches lost: _____

Present hips: _____

Inches lost: _____

Present upper arms: _____

Inches lost: _____

Present thighs: _____

Inches lost: _____

When you look back over the past week . . .

How do you feel? How is your energy level?

_____

_____

_____

How did you sleep this week?

_____

_____

_____

Were the first few days hard? On what day did you start feeling better?

_____

_____

_____

Did you have cravings this week? Was it difficult to resist them?

_____

_____

_____

What other challenges did you face this week? How did you deal with them?

_____

_____

_____

Did you skip any meals?

_____
_____
_____

Did you eat three cups of vegetables?

_____
_____
_____

Did you take your supplements?

_____
_____
_____

Did you drink a minimum of eight 8-ounce glasses of water?

_____
_____
_____

Did you eat any forbidden foods?

_____
_____
_____

If so, how did they make you feel?

_____
_____
_____

And were you able to get right back on track?

_____
_____
_____

Did anyone make comments about your being on the ANA? How did you respond?

_____
_____
_____

What strategies are working for you? What changes do you need to make?

_____
_____
_____

Are you happy with your progress?

_____
_____
_____

7 ▸ Your Second Week on Atkins

One thing I noticed right off the bat was how often my teenage son and I had been eating on the run. Before Atkins, we'd just throw something in the microwave. Suddenly I was forced to fix meals to follow the program. That actually turned out to be a blessing. We'd sit down together at the dinner table and really communicate. This has really brought us together.

—Jan Baumer, lost 19 pounds

You're off and running in your second week on Atkins. You've found a routine, you're feeling full of energy and any of those pesky symptoms you felt during the first few days are a thing of the past. You are ready to step up your fitness regimen or begin exercising if you have not been active lately. You are feeling in control of your appetite instead of vice versa. Best of all, the fat is coming off—and that's according to the tape measure, your new friend the scale and the way your clothes are starting to feel less snug. Okay, is this an accurate reflection of what's going on with you?

If it is, congratulations! You are among the many fortunate folks for whom the Atkins Nutritional Approach™ (ANA) will, in all likelihood, banish your unwanted pounds. And, if so, keep doing exactly what you are doing.

If not, however, don't despair. First, double-check your measurements. Some people lose inches without losing pounds. (This can happen in any phase of Atkins.) If that's not the case, it just means you're among the small percentage of people whose bodies are somewhat resistant to shedding pounds, a condition commonly referred to as *metabolic resistance*. Like life, it's not fair, but we can help you overcome most of the reasons for this annoying tendency.

► Reasons for Resistance

Resistance to weight loss can occur for a number of reasons. Some can be influenced by changes in behavior or lifestyle. For example, if you are eating too much, you can learn to moderate your portions. If you are sedentary, you can find an exercise regimen that you enjoy and that suits your lifestyle. Individuals with very high insulin levels are likely to be slow starters, meaning that they may lose very little weight (or none) until they have controlled carbohydrates for a longer period of time than people with more normal insulin levels.

Another possibility: You may lose slowly in the week before your menstrual period. Cravings may also be aggravated during this time. Just be patient. Weight loss is likely to speed up once you have finished your menses.

Solving other problems, such as an underactive thyroid or use of medications that either make you gain weight or slow weight loss are more complex, but in concert with your doctor, you can seek solutions.

Then there are the things you simply cannot do anything about: Genetics and age are obviously beyond your control. So is hormonal status—menopause and perimenopause typically slow a woman's metabolism— or a sluggish thyroid. In such cases, you need to readjust your expectations. You may never get down to the weight you were as a younger person, or it may take you longer than you had originally hoped.

Another common reason for your body to resist weight loss is a history of going on and off diets, known as yo-yo dieting. When you get into a pattern of repeatedly losing and gaining weight, your body becomes adept at protecting its fat stores by slowing down your metabolism.

MEDICATIONS THAT INTERFERE
WITH WEIGHT LOSS

If you're having trouble losing weight, don't overlook the contents of your medicine cabinet. Certainly, metabolic abnormalities such as insulin resistance can make it difficult to lose weight, but far more people are stalled in their pound-paring efforts because of prescription medications they are taking. **(Note: Under no circumstances should you decrease your dosage or eliminate a prescription medication without your physician's supervision.)** Some common culprits include:

- **Antidepressants**, particularly those in the SSRI (selective serotonin reuptake inhibitors) category, are serious offenders when it comes to presenting obstacles to weight loss. Common side effects of these SSRIs, such as anxiety, sleeplessness, nervousness and headaches, actually create carbohydrate cravings. Many older psychotropic drugs (tricyclic antidepressants) also are known to cause weight gain.
- **Estrogen** and most synthetic hormone replacement therapies (HRTs), including birth control pills, can cause weight gain and inhibit weight loss. Many standard hormones create an estrogen dominance, or insulin resistance, which can interfere with weight loss.

- **Drugs for high blood pressure**, especially diuretics and the drugs known as beta-blockers, can make your body extremely resistant to weight loss. As you lose weight, your blood pressure often improves; your doctor will have to reduce your dosage so that you do not over-dose on blood-pressure medication.

Talk to your doctor about alternatives to these and other medications, such as steroids, NSAIDs and statins, that might be interfering with your weight loss. Again, never adjust or taper off drugs without consulting your physician.

▶ Dealing with Sluggish Weight Loss

If you're facing less than steady weight loss at this point, it just means that your body is a bit slow to re-lease its fat stores and your weight loss will likely be more gradual. If you are a slow loser, you may also ex-perience frustrating stalls, when the pounds simply re-fuse to budge at all. Be patient. Don't let it get you down, and by all means, don't give up! Extreme meta-bolic resistance may require you to make the following small adjustments:

- **Get your body moving.** The first thing you should do is heed the ANA prescription for exercise (see Chapter 8). As long as you're feeling well and no longer in the throes of any withdrawal symptoms, incorporate a new physical activity into your day. ANA followers from all walks of life report that exercise jump-starts weight loss—as can switching from one type of exercise to a new one.

- **Make sure that you are not consuming more carbs than you think**. Carbs are in many foods that you may not immediately think of, such as salad dressings. Also measure your portions until you can learn to eyeball them. (See "Visualizing Portion Sizes" on page 104.) You may inadvertently be eating larger portions and therefore more grams of Net Carbs than you think you are. It is also a good idea not to eat while engaging in another activity such as watching television or driving. It is obviously harder to keep track of what is going in your mouth when your focus is elsewhere. Eating in front of the TV, for example, may lead to making poor food choices.

- **Cut out higher carb foods**. The next thing you need to do is omit the handful of higher carb foods on the "Acceptable Induction Foods" list—avocado, olives, lime and lemon juice, and cream or sour cream—and watch that you are not eating too much protein or too little fat, or both. You can also cut back on your serving sizes of cheese. Low carb alternative foods also can pose a problem for some stubborn losers. You may need to cut down, say, from a whole low carb protein bar to half of one. Also look for "hidden carbs" you may not be aware of.

- **Cut back on your protein consumption**. When you eat too much protein at one sitting, some of it will convert to blood sugar, which will interfere with fat burning. Keep portion sizes reasonable, and eat smaller, more frequent meals. You should feel satisfied, but not stuffed, after a meal. Making yourself eat more slowly can also help you judge when you are full. If you are not sure how much to eat because you have been overeating for years, try eating less than you have been accustomed to at a meal. After 30 minutes, if you are no longer hungry, you will begin to notice the difference between habit and real hunger. Eventually you should learn when to stop eating, which will promote weight loss.

- **Eat at least three meals a day**. Skipping meals or going too long between meals (you should not go more than six waking hours) will cause your blood sugar level to drop, which can make you tired, jittery and hungry. Regular meals and low carb snacks keep your blood sugar on an even keel, which makes you less likely to give in to your cravings for carbs or to overeat at your next meal. The best way to avoid overeating is to never let yourself get ravenous.

- **If you are constipated, deal with it**. (See "Coping with Constipation" on pages 96–99.) Not only will you retain weight, being constipated makes you feel sluggish, so you are less apt to get out and exercise.

- **Be sure you are drinking at least eight 8-ounce glasses of water a day**. Not only does drinking plenty of water combat constipation, it allows you to distinguish between hunger and thirst. Your body may signal that it wants more food, when it really needs water. Adequate hydration is necessary for the proper functioning of chemical reactions in the body. Dehydration will make them less efficient and can slow weight loss.

- **Don't overconsume artificial sweeteners**. Each packet contains almost a full gram of carbohydrates, so if you are using five a day, you are squandering one-quarter of your carb allowance. Limit yourself to no more than three packets a day. Some people find that using sweeteners makes it harder for them to break their carbohydrate addiction. If you still crave sweets in the second week on Induction, eliminate all sweeteners and see if cravings diminish and weight loss picks up.

- **Cut out caffeine**. If you are addicted to caffeine and have not switched to decaf coffee, do so now. Excessive caffeine in the form of coffee, tea and cola drinks may be affecting your blood sugar levels, making you crave sweets.

THE THYROID GLAND AND SLUGGISH WEIGHT LOSS

An underactive thyroid—the medical condition known as hypothyroidism—can slow your metabolism and get in the way of weight loss. Among other things, your thyroid gland regulates your body temperature. In fact, sensitivity to cold is one of the first signs that you may have a sluggish thyroid. Other symptoms include weight gain or the inability to lose weight, hair loss, fatigue and lethargy, depression, dry skin, chronic constipation, poor nails, poor memory and elevated cholesterol levels.

Like other hormones, thyroid production naturally diminishes slightly with age; easily 25 percent of adults suffer from low thyroid function. The swings of estrogen production in perimenopause or menopause can also throw off thyroid function, as can some medications such as birth control pills and lithium, among others.

If you suspect that you might have an underactive thyroid, talk to your doctor, who will likely perform blood tests—specifically free T3, free T4 and

TSH. These tests evaluate your production of thyroid hormones T4 (also known as thyroxine) and T3 (your body converts T4 to T3), as well as another hormone called TSH (thyroid-stimulating hormone), which is produced by your pituitary gland.

The bottom line is that weight loss is a very individual matter and each person will respond differently to consuming only 20 grams of Net Carbs a day. Because everyone's situation and metabolism is different, the ANA is designed to be individualized to your tastes and needs. If you are not happy with your results, rather than thinking of abandoning the plan, make adjustments until it begins working for you. If you have to cut back on carbs to launch your weight loss, you can add them back in a week or two, once your body has made the shift and is cruising along in fat-burning mode. So if you are not losing at 20 grams of Net Carbs a day, cut back to 15 for a few days. This would mean eating only three cups of salads and eliminating other carb foods. (Conversely, if you added back a serving or two of carbs to relieve symptoms, return to 20 grams of Net Carbs when your body has adjusted to this new way of eating.)

The first two weeks on Induction were hard. I was irritable and sleepy all the time. I had no energy. But once I broke through my sugar addiction, the weight started melting off and I started feeling great—better than I ever had. I began walking at lunchtime, which really helped speed up my weight loss and was a great stress reliever. I'd walk for about an hour and then come back to my desk and snack on chicken or precooked Swedish meatballs, beef jerky or nuts. Eventually, I worked up to hiking, which brought me to my first goal weight of 240. Once I was down to that weight, I could bike at lunchtime. Now, at 205 with 25 pounds to go, I bike 22 miles at lunchtime three days a week and go surfing and kayaking on the other days!

—*James Guilbeaux, lost 100 pounds*

If you haven't yet completed Week Two of Induction at this point, do not move on to the following section until you have.

► Decision Time

You've done it! You've completed the first two weeks of the ANA and you're passed the hurdles of the transition, you're burning fat and feeling great. That's why the two-week marker is a logical time for evaluation.

So turn to page 127 now, fill out your "Where I Am Today" sheet for Day 14, answer the questions and then turn back to this page.

The first decision to make is an obvious one: Should you continue with the ANA? The second decision to make is: Should you move to the next phase, Ongoing Weight Loss (OWL)? Some of you, especially people with relatively modest weight-loss goals—say, 20 to 30 pounds—will be ready to move on to OWL. Others will choose to stay on Induction. If you have a lot of weight to lose, you can safely continue on Induction for six months or more. You can also choose to move to OWL if you prefer. It's up to you. Chapter 9 will help you make this decision.

Note: You should not stay on Induction until you are at your goal weight. It is essential that you move through the various phases at appropriate times. This is key to finding your tolerance for carb intake, which is essential to success on Lifetime Maintenance and establishing better overall eating habits.

► Should You Continue on the ANA?

First, let's consider the question of whether or not you'll continue doing Atkins altogether. We think the answer is obvious, but perhaps it isn't to you. If you're thinking of stopping the ANA, we strongly urge you to reconsider.

Let's look at four of the reasons people give for not continuing, one by one:

1. I have lost enough weight.
2. I have *not* lost enough weight.

3. I miss bread, cereal, fruit, potatoes and other high carb foods too much.
4. My friends or family tell me it's not good to do Atkins long term.

Let's look at these excuses:

1. If you have lost all the weight you wanted to lose in just two weeks, good for you. You may feel you can now go it on your own, just watching your carbs. While this is where you'll eventually find yourself when you reach Lifetime Maintenance, experience tells us that two weeks is not long enough to habituate to an entirely new way of eating. It is almost inevitable that you will gradually sink back into your old way of eating. You won't have made a firm lifestyle change and the pounds will reappear. Advancing through the other three phases of Atkins and gradually returning most carbohydrate foods to your menus will teach you the good eating habits that are absolutely essential to maintain your new weight long term.

2. Maybe you're one of the people who didn't lose the amount of weight you had hoped to shed. Do you go immediately to thinking, "Oh, here's another diet that doesn't work for me"? You've heard of all these people shedding pounds like mad on Atkins and you're frustrated that it didn't work that way for you. Please believe us when we say you

are not alone. Or don't take our word for it—go to the Atkins Web site (*www.atkins.com*) and you'll find success stories written by people who were as resistant to losing weight as you are, maybe more so. You may also find low carb forums on the Internet, where you can "chat" with people who have faced the same obstacles you face. Consider whether giving up too quickly and returning to your old ways is a behavior pattern you have exhibited in the past.

It may take you a little more time than other people you know, but the weight *will* come off if you stick to the plan. Having an Atkins buddy who is your sex, roughly your age and has a similar amount to lose can also be enormously helpful. So too can enlisting your spouse. Just remember that two individuals never lose at exactly the same rate, so don't expect your progress to mirror your buddy's.

Another thing to consider: Eating this way has two purposes. You must not forget that weight loss is just one component of the ANA; increased health—and with it, decreased risk for disease—is the other paramount objective.

3. If you are still craving carbs, there are several possibilities:

- You are cheating, and thereby stimulating your blood sugar roller coaster to want more carbs as your blood sugar level drops.

- You are not cheating, but are consuming the entire 20 grams of Net Carbs at one meal. If you have a history of unstable blood sugar, this may be too much at one time, and you will need to spread your allotment of carbs over the course of the day.

- You are not actively cheating, but are consuming "hidden" carbs in foods you are unaware have them. These usually lurk in prepared foods such as canned and dried soups, salad dressings, sauces, gravies, frozen vegetables with sauces that contain cornstarch, fillers such as milk solids and even sugar. Condiments that often contain sugar in one form or another include barbecue sauce, ketchup, sandwich spreads, and teriyaki sauce. If you are using "diet" mayonnaise or sour cream or other "diet" products, a look at the list of ingredients will often show you that fat has been replaced with sugar for flavor. Become vigilant about reading Nutrition Facts panels. Another good rule of thumb is to avoid all low fat or diet foods unless they are specifically described as low in carbs and have no added sugar.

- Your cravings are not physical cravings caused by unstable blood sugar but are ingrained habits you are not willing to leave behind. You may need a sweet sensation that can be achieved with low carb alternatives.

Until you actually get into fat-burning mode, which has an appetite-suppressing effect, you may have trouble staying away from your old food companions, those very ones that got you into trouble in the first place.

Also remember that Induction is the most restrictive phase of Atkins. As you move through the increasingly liberal phases that conclude with Lifetime Maintenance, you will be gradually and carefully adding back nutrient-dense carbohydrate foods. In Ongoing Weight Loss, one of the first foods you can reintroduce is berries. By the time you are in Pre-Maintenance, you will likely be able to add back whole grains, other fruits and even the occasional potato.

4. If your results are good but you are under pressure from friends and family—or even your physician—to stop doing Atkins, review "From Sabotage to Support," on pages 44–45, and "Talking to Your Doctor About Atkins," pages 49–50. Also check out the studies on pages 349–352, which should soothe you and any Atkins detractors. Then think about your weight-loss results and how much better you feel after two weeks doing Atkins. Sometimes you just have to listen to your own inner voice—and your body—and not the din of well-meaning but not well-informed people around you.

Whatever your reason for considering abandoning the program, we would urge you to reconsider for all of the aforementioned reasons. In time, you will begin to love the controlled carb lifestyle and all that it contributes to your life.

► **Food for Thought**

Fill out your vital statistics and answer the questions below on Day 14 of Induction. Compare your results with your first two sets.

"DAY 14: WHERE I AM TODAY"

Date you started doing Atkins: _____
Present weight: _____
Pounds lost: _____
Goal weight: _____
Present clothing size: _____
Goal clothing size: _____
Present chest: _____
Inches lost: _____
Present waist: _____
Inches lost: _____
Present hips: _____
Inches lost: _____
Present upper arms: _____
Inches lost: _____
Present thighs: _____
Inches lost: _____

When you look back over the past week . . .

How has your mood been?

_____

_____

_____

How has your energy level been?

_____

_____

_____

Did you exercise each day?

_____

_____

_____

Did you increase your time spent exercising this week?

_____

_____

_____

Did you increase your exercise intensity this week?

_____

_____

_____

Did you eat any vegetables that you have not regularly eaten in the past week?

_____
_____
_____

How did you sleep this week?

_____
_____
_____

Did you have cravings this week? Was it difficult to resist them?

_____
_____
_____

What other challenges did you face this week? How did you deal with them?

_____
_____
_____

Did anyone make comments about your being on the ANA? How did you respond?

_____
_____
_____

What strategies are working for you? What changes do you need to make?

_____

_____

_____

Are you happy with your progress?

_____

_____

_____

8 ▶ Move It to Lose It

As a high school principal and former athlete who had been promoting fitness and good health my whole life, I should never have let myself get to the 323 pounds I was at age 38. Thanks to doing Atkins, I'm down to 218, my waist went from 52 to 38 inches and my wife introduces me as her "new boyfriend." I feel better now than I have in 18 years. Now I'm back to an hour's workout every morning that includes the treadmill, stationary bike and weight training. My biggest problem is that I have to keep buying new pants!

—Tim Johnston, lost 105 pounds

Once you've made the switch to fat burning and are feeling on top of the world, it's time to harness that newfound energy and use it to advance your quest to be slimmer and healthier. Doing Atkins has turned many a couch potato into an exercise buff. This is due to the great Atkins Nutritional Approach™ (ANA)-and-exercise combo deal: The ANA helps you lose

weight and gives you energy, which makes you want to
exercise, which helps you lose more weight and gives
you more energy, and so on! It's a win-win proposi-
tion. Moreover, if you don't exercise regularly while
controlling your carbs, you're not doing the ANA
properly and you're shortchanging yourself in several
important ways.

**Note: Consult with your physician before begin-
ning any exercise program; if you have any pre-
existing cardiovascular disease or have been leading
a very sedentary lifestyle, a consultation with a
cardiologist is imperative.**

► Why Exercise Is <u>Not</u> a Choice

To reiterate: Along with your new eating plan, you
absolutely *must* incorporate physical activity into your
daily life. One of the misconceptions about the ANA is
that you do not have to exercise. Not true. Exercise is
an integral part of Atkins and you must not ignore it.
Exercising every day will:

- Increase your fat burning and weight loss (even
  when you are at rest!)
- Tone and strengthen your muscles
- Help keep skin from sagging as fat comes off
- Keep your energy level up
- Help you sleep better
- Improve your mood

- Reduce your risk of injuries
- Help ward off diabetes, heart disease, stroke, cancer and virtually every life-threatening disease out there
- Help maintain bone mass and decrease the risk of osteoporosis for both men and women

At this stage, you may be focusing primarily on benefit number one: increasing fat burning and weight loss. Eventually, the other reasons will be compelling unto themselves. In the meantime, let us explain further how exercise will complement your eating plan in helping you to shed pounds.

Exercise of any kind helps you build, or at least maintain, muscle mass. And weight-bearing exercise, in particular, builds muscle mass. Many overweight people avoid weight training because they fear they'll get bigger muscles and look even larger. This is a complete misconception that we'll go into a bit later. For now, we want you to understand that building muscle mass will help you lose fat. A quick warning: When you're building muscle, there's a chance you'll stop showing weight loss on your scale—or you might even see a small weight gain. That's because muscle is denser than fat. But you will see the difference in your body and the way your clothes fit. More important, muscle requires more energy from your body every day than fat does. In other words, by increasing muscle mass, you will burn more calories even when you're standing still.

This means that exercising helps you lose weight three different ways:

1. The obvious one—you burn more calories during exercise.
2. After you finish your workout, your metabolism stays elevated for a period of time—during which you're burning more calories than usual.
3. Once you've begun to increase muscle mass, your metabolism is cranked up a notch, 24/7, even when you're standing in line at the bank!

Now we're sure you'll agree: Exercise is a no-brainer. So let's get going and figure out what you need to do to start moving and shaking that body.

▶ Make Exercise Your Ally

If you haven't exercised before or have gotten out of the habit, first talk to your doctor. If he or she gives you the green light, start with a walk. Don't overanalyze it, don't dread it, and don't wait until you've bought new sneakers. Just do it. Strap on your watch and head out the door. Walk for 15 minutes and see how it makes you feel. (**Hint:** Exercise first thing in the morning instead of fooling yourself into thinking you will do it later. You never know what distractions will arise.) Gradually increase your time and intensity, with a goal of being active for a total of one hour a day. Don't roll your eyes! This can be broken up throughout the day into a half hour walk, a 15-minute bike ride and 15 minutes of dancing, aerobics, jogging in place or anything else that gets your heart rate up. You can hit a tennis ball against a wall, walk up and down your stairs a few times or do some brisk housecleaning.

Get information on exercises you can do in the water or in a chair—great, low-impact ways to break into becoming physically active again. It's important that you start slowly and learn how to stretch, warm up and cool down to avoid injury. When taking on a new exercise or sport, consult with a certified fitness professional to learn proper form and technique. Otherwise, you may sprain, twist or strain something and derail your program altogether.

It doesn't matter what you do, just that you do it. And so the most important thing is to choose the activities that you enjoy the most—or hate the least. As you become more fit and look for challenges beyond walking, a whole world of alternatives unfolds. Here's a quick list to get you thinking:

- **Bicycling:** You can easily get your heart rate up on a bike without putting stress on your joints. If you have access to a gym, you can choose from a regular stationary bike or a *recumbent* bike, which is easier on your back and bottom.

- **Running:** Running is not for everyone. If you are still significantly overweight or have knee problems or other skeletal injuries, it's definitely not for you. Still, running is more challenging than walking, and for many people it's a logical and thrilling progression from walking. How can you tell if you're ready to run? If you can walk 45 minutes quickly, without rest, you're probably ready to pick up the pace. Start by finding a treadmill or a local high-school or college track. Outdoor tracks are usually about a quarter mile around, closed to traffic and have an ideal surface. Walk a few laps (or about 15 minutes on a treadmill) to warm up, then try one lap (or two to three minutes) of jogging at an easy pace. Or, on a track, jog the straightaway but then walk the curves at each end of the track.

- **Swimming:** If you have arthritis, knee pain or a lot of weight to lose, swimming is ideal. The water supports your body, giving you the freedom to move in an impact-free environment. If swimming on your own doesn't thrill you, try water aerobics classes (check your local YMCA or YWCA or health club). Because swimming uses so many muscle groups at the same time, it is a very efficient way to exercise.

- **Elliptical trainers:** You'll find these machines in most well-equipped gyms. An elliptical trainer moves each of your legs in an oval- or ellipse-shaped motion. Some models have handlebars that you push and pull in sequence with the footpads for an additional upper-body workout. This very low-impact motion is smooth and comfortable—a good choice for someone prone to knee or other joint pain.

- **Steppers and stair climbers:** These are definitely not for everyone. Stepping machines can aggravate knee problems and they're easy to misuse. If you make any of the common mistakes—leaning on the console, letting the pedals touch the ground or hopping like a bunny from one pedal to the other—you aren't getting much benefit, and the strain on your wrists may actually increase your risk for carpal tunnel syndrome. Still, when used correctly, they offer a simple, effective workout. These machines can provide quite an aerobic challenge and should be approached with care by those less fit or not accustomed to stair climbing.

- **Rowing machines:** If you have access to a rower, try it! These machines work your trunk muscles and arms—a rarity in the leg-centric cardio room—while getting your heart rate up. If you're comfortable on the rowing machine, use it to break up the monotony of other cardio exercises.

- **Aerobics or dance classes:** Jazz Dance, World Beat, Hip Hop, kick boxing, you name it. Take whatever appeals to you, but remember: Just because you're in a group doesn't mean you have to keep pace. Do what's right for you. If you need to slow down or modify a move, do it. Conversely, if the class isn't challenging enough for you, pick up your pace.

- **Yoga:** Many people think practicing yoga is primarily about stretching and stress relief. It can be, but depending on the type of yoga you do and how you approach it, it can also be an incredible—even tough—anaerobic and aerobic workout. Some popular forms of yoga—Power Yoga, Ashtanga and Bikram yoga, for example—are vigorous routines that raise your heart rate and build muscle. What's great about yoga is that it also increases flexibility, helps prevent injury and calms the mind. And it requires no special clothing or equipment. Yoga classes are offered everywhere these days and, again, books and videos abound if you prefer to do it on your own.

- **Pilates:** This unique type of exercise takes place on floor mats and also on apparatus specifically designed for Pilates. It requires a trained instructor and, whether you take group classes or individual instruction, can be an expensive endeavor. Like yoga, Pilates stretches and strengthens the body while also employing focused breathing. It is known especially for training and building the muscles of the body's "core," or trunk, including the abdominals and lower back. Pilates devotees say it is the best all-over body workout you can find.

- **Resistance bands:** An extremely simple and effective way to work your muscles, resistance bands can be used almost anywhere. They're also standard equipment now in most gyms. Like giant rubber bands, often made of tubing with foam handles, resistance bands can be used to strengthen virtually any muscle in your body. You can buy them at fitness stores or online in different sizes and levels of resistance. Then look for instructions in books, videos or from a fitness trainer at your local health club or YMCA or YWCA.

- **Chair exercises:** This is an ideal way for an older, weaker or very overweight individual to begin a fitness program. Even in a chair, you can strengthen your muscles, help prevent joint and muscle stiffness and keep your body limber— as well as reduce stress—by stretching while seated. There are specific exercises for the neck, shoulders, arms, back, stomach and legs. Videos depicting chair exercises are readily available.

➤ The Yin and Yang of Working Out

You probably know that there are two types of exercise: **aerobic** and **anaerobic**. They are equally important and they complement each other. It's generally smart, when making the switch from a very sedentary lifestyle, to begin with aerobic exercise and then incorporate anaerobic gradually.

1. **Aerobic** activity is anything that increases your heart rate and makes you consume more oxygen. While the word may bring to mind women in leotards bouncing to loud music, activities such as walking, golf, horseback riding, Ping-Pong and even ballroom dancing fall into the category of aerobic exercise. They may only moderately increase your heart rate but, for someone who is starting from nothing, there can be a tremendous improvement. Once you begin doing something physical on a regular basis, you will feel such a difference that you'll be hooked. Stiffness or soreness will abate, breathing will improve and those relaxing endorphins will be released into your bloodstream, giving you a subtle, natural high.

How much aerobic exercise do you need? As we previously stated, you should shoot for one hour a day, every day. However, if you're starting from zero, you should begin with as little as 10 minutes a day, after checking with a doctor.

How intense does your workout need to be? You can track your own heart rate or buy a heart-rate monitor to keep yourself in your target heart-rate zone (see page 141), or you can monitor your own exertion by paying attention to how your body feels. Are you feeling a little out of breath? You should be huffing a little but not gasping for air. Can you talk? You should be able to speak in short sentences but not hold long conversations. Are you working hard? You should feel as though you're pushing yourself but not as though you're about to keel over.

FIND YOUR TARGET HEART-RATE ZONE

Subtract your age from 220, and then take 60 percent and 70 percent of that number. Mathematically, the formulas are:

(220 − your age) × .60 = lower end of your zone

(220 − your age) × .70 = higher end of your zone

So a sample calculation for a 58-year-old woman would be:

220 − 58 = 162 × .60 = 97
220 − 58 = 162 × .70 = 113

This woman should keep her pulse between 97 and 113 beats per minute while exercising. Very overweight people should be especially careful, because they may reach the high end of their zone quite quickly. People who are already fit may be able to go higher than 70 percent.

---

2. **Anaerobic** activity is the other side of the exercise equation. While you can and should do some aerobic exercise every day of the week, anaerobic exercise should be rotated between the upper and lower

body to give muscle tissue a day to repair between workouts. Alternatively, you could do total body workouts every other day.

Anaerobic exercise is any type of physical activity that is not significantly aerobic. This includes exercise that builds muscle mass, such as weight lifting and resistance training. Don't assume this requires a complete set of free weights or Nautilus machines, however. Push-ups, sit-ups, or lifting cans of tomatoes are all legitimate anaerobic exercises. As we mentioned before, another misconception about this type of exercise is that it will bulk you up, leaving you with big, bulging body parts. Any bodybuilder will tell you that it takes more than three times a week of moderate weight lifting to get those kinds of bodies. If you work hard and never miss a weight-training day, you still won't look like them. What you'll see is a beautiful, subtle sculpting taking place under your skin that will change the way clothes hang on you, the way you hold yourself when you walk, and the way you feel walking up a flight of stairs.

In addition to building muscle mass—which, as we discussed, helps you burn more calories, even at rest—weight-bearing exercise is very important for protecting and strengthening your bones, which lose density as you get older. Along with getting enough calcium (which many adults do not, but on Atkins you will), weight-bearing exercise is the best way to prevent osteoporosis.

One note of caution: With anaerobic exercise, it

is vitally important that you use correct form and technique. Consult a professional—whether it's a fitness trainer at your local YMCA or YWCA or a good exercise book or video—to learn what to do and what not to do, so that you don't end up with a back, shoulder, hip or groin injury on your first go-round.

By now, you are probably convinced that regular exercise is a very good thing, and you should have some ideas about which activities you are going to pursue. We hope you have at least the beginnings of a plan in place that will get you exercising most days of the week. We also hope this plan will eventually include weight or resistance training along with aerobic activity. Now it's only fair that we give you some tips on how to get more exercise into your life with the least amount of trouble. And how to make sure you stick with it.

► Ten Tips for Getting Your Workouts In

1. **Ride, run or walk to work.** If you have a shower at work, this is a great way to start the day and make the most of your time.
2. **Work out at lunchtime.** A midday exercise break helps boost energy and makes the afternoon fly by.
3. **Exercise in front of the television**. This way, you are less likely to put off a workout so that you can watch your favorite show. Watching

the tube can become a reason to work out, rather than a deterrent.

4. **Exercise with friends or coworkers.** If you use your exercise time as a way to socialize, you can accomplish two goals at once. Group workouts are also a great way to meet new people with a shared interest, so check out local running or walking clubs or group exercise classes for times that fit your schedule.

5. **Get up early.** Morning is your friend. With practice, predawn workouts can become found hours.

6. **Exercise at home.** If you have a workout setup at home or use exercise videos, you don't need to find the added motivation and additional time to get yourself dressed and out of the house.

7. **Make a plan.** Following a schedule is a powerful tool in the battle to stay on target. Look at the week in advance and pick your time slots carefully. Remember that it is always safer to start the day with your workout than to plan on getting to it later.

8. **Make a date.** Try the buddy system. If you commit to meeting someone for an early workout, chances are you will show up—at least after the first time you sleep in and your buddy plays up the guilt factor.

9. **Exercise before you go home.** If you normally drive home during rush hour and there is a way to exercise near your workplace, you

may be able to avoid wasting time in traffic along with the pitfalls of procrastination.

10. **Keep your priorities straight.** The benefits of exercise do not outweigh the importance of experiencing what is most valuable in life: time spent with friends and family. Use these tips to maximize your time with the people who matter most. In the long run, exercise may just give you several extra years to spend with those very people.

We think we've made the case for exercise pretty clear—and we've provided some basic how-to's. Now the ball is in your court: It's completely up to you. Don't let another day go by without a brisk walk, at the very least. Do it for your body, for your heart, for the people you love and, most of all, for yourself.

► Food for Thought

You've learned why you need to exercise. Answer the following questions to understand how you can make it a regular part of your life—and even something you begin to enjoy.

In the past, have you had a bad "relationship" with exercise? Do you hate exercise?

_____

_____

_____

Of all the types of physical activity you have tried or heard about, choose three that appeal to you the most (or are the least *unappealing* to you). What equipment, location and preparation would be needed for you to do each of these activities?

_____

_____

_____

Have you ever exercised with a buddy or a group? Did you find the time passed more quickly than when you've exercised alone?

_____

_____

_____

What is the hardest part of exercising for you: boredom, exertion, pain, embarrassment, finding time, making yourself go, or something else?

_____

_____

_____

What is one thing you can do this week to make it easier to exercise? (This could be anything from calling a friend to schedule a walk to putting your sneakers and exercise clothes by your bed so you have to put them on when you first wake up.)

_____

_____

_____

Did you know that exercise keeps your metabolism elevated even after you've stopped moving?

_____

_____

_____

Did you know that increasing your muscle mass also increases your permanent at-rest metabolic rate—which makes it easier to lose weight and keep it off?

_____

_____

_____

9 ► Stay Put or Move On?

> *My biggest challenge was avoiding temptation during the holidays. Although my family was behind me, there were so many high carb foods around that I gave in—only on Christmas. And then I felt so fatigued the next day that I knew I'd never cheat again. I've lost 56 pounds so far, but have decided to stick to 20 grams of Net Carbs a day for now because my goal is to lose another 34 pounds. My energy level has skyrocketed and my daily migraines and heartburn have disappeared. Even my skin looks better.*
>
> *—Jason Shepherd, lost 56 pounds*

The issue we're about to explore—whether you should stay on Induction or move on to Ongoing Weight Loss (OWL)—may present a simple answer for you. Do you feel great on Induction and have a lot more of those pesky pounds to lose? Are you finding Induction increasingly easy to do and enjoying the foods you're eating? Many people decide to stay on Induction for these reasons. Some people feel safer at this point sticking with a more confined menu, fearing that if they begin to give themselves more choices, they will stray and fall off the edge. Another important reason to stay on Induction and continue losing relatively quickly is a medical condition that makes weight reduction a priority.

In addition, you may be someone whose body is especially resistant to weight loss, meaning the pounds will come off relatively slowly. You'll know if you fall into this category after reading Chapter 7. If you do, you can benefit from remaining on Induction because it gives you time to correct metabolic imbalances that may have developed over time. These include insulin resistance, blood sugar imbalances, carbohydrate addictions and allergies. Once these metabolic imbalances are corrected, your weight loss may speed up.

The good news is that you can stay on Induction for the time being—so long as you eat carbohydrate foods full of nutrients and take your supplementary vitamins and minerals (including essential oils).

That said, it is worth repeating that the Atkins Nutritional Approach™ (ANA) is a four-phase program. Induction is not the way you should be eating for the rest of your life. People who stay on Induction until they have reached their goal weight sometimes have trouble transitioning into Lifetime Maintenance. They have not learned which foods they can handle and which they need to moderate or eliminate. That is a key reason for the phased approach.

NIBBLE ON NUTS

If you do decide to stay on Induction, your reward is that you can now add an ounce of delicious nuts and seeds to your daily intake and see how you do. Nuts contain protein, fat and carbohydrates, but a significant portion of the carbs is fiber. Of course, you need to count the grams of Net Carbs in your daily tally. Most nuts are fine, but macadamias have the highest ratio of fat to carbohydrate. Cashews and peanuts are slightly higher in carbs so it's best to stick with macadamias, almonds, pecans, hazelnuts, pine nuts and walnuts at the start. Don't overlook pumpkin seeds, sunflower seeds, and sesame seeds, all of which add a delicious crunch to salads and cooked veggies.

These little powerhouses are also densely packed with nutrients. Almonds are a rich source of calcium. Almonds, sunflower seeds and hazelnuts are particularly rich in vitamin E. Nuts also provide a long list of other nutrients, including niacin, vitamin B6, folic acid, magnesium, zinc, copper and potassium, plus a number of phytochemicals, including many antioxidants.

You can also use ground nuts and seeds in lieu of bread crumbs before baking or sautéing chicken breasts, veal scallops or fish fillets. Like all good things, nuts and seeds should be eaten in moderation.

Numerous studies have shown that regular consumption of nuts and seeds minimizes your risk for coronary heart disease. People who eat nuts regularly are less likely to have a heart attack than people who do not consume nuts and oil-containing seeds. It's the monounsaturated fat in nuts that makes them so good for your health. People on low fat diets often eliminate nuts—and with them a powerful source of omega fatty acids and other nutrients.

Be sure to avoid nuts that have been coated with sugar or honey. One last caveat about nuts and seeds: Like chips, they are notoriously easy to keep eating once you start. Never eat directly from a large bag or can. Instead, portion out your daily allowance and eat only that.

In a Nutshell

Here's how to estimate a one-ounce portion of the following nuts and seeds:

- 24 almonds
- 18 cashews
- 20 filberts (hazelnuts)
- 10–12 medium macadamias
- 28 shelled peanuts
- 20 pecan halves
- 157 pine nuts (pignoli)
- 47 pistachios
- 14 walnut halves
- 1 tablespoon pumpkin seeds
- 1 medium-size handful sesame seeds
- 3 tablespoons of shelled sunflower seeds

➤ When It's Time to Move to OWL

How can you be sure you're ready to make the leap from Induction to Ongoing Weight Loss (OWL)? There are several reasons to begin forging ahead:

- **You're getting close to your goal weight.** You may have already lost a good chunk of the weight you have to lose. If that's the case, it is important that you slow things down a bit. You need to gradually adjust to what will become your new way of eating—and to your new, slimmer body! By stepping up to OWL, you begin the gradual move toward your individualized level of carbohydrate consumption.

- **You're bored on Induction.** This is also a good reason to move on. Boredom can lead to being tempted to cheat, something to avoid at all costs. Of course, you need to remember that moving on to OWL is not a license to go wild. It just means you can begin, ever so slowly, increasing your healthy carb intake—one week at a time. The Rules of OWL are outlined in Part Four of this book, along with those for subsequent phases.

- **You want to relax your food choices.** In this case, the more liberal phase of OWL will likely be the solution you are seeking. If a longer period of time until you get to your goal weight is the trade-off you're willing to make to have a wider array of foods to eat, go for it. The decision is yours alone and is another example of how much individualization is possible when doing Atkins.

- **You're developing a "quick fix" mentality.** When people learn that they can lose weight quickly, as they do during Induction, they sometimes take their newfound ability to lose weight for granted. They don't think in terms of the necessary lifetime commitment to the ANA. The results of this thinking are yo-yo dieting and metabolic resistance to weight loss. While OWL may likely slow your rate of weight loss, this is not a bad thing. The slower the progress, the greater the chances that you will permanently change bad habits over the long term.

ONGOING CHALLENGES

If you decide to move on to OWL, you need to be aware that as you increase your carb consumption, the wonderful appetite-suppressing effect of burning fat begins to diminish somewhat and you will need to rely increasingly on willpower. Psychological addictions are harder to break than cravings caused by blood sugar swings. You'll need to develop tactics to avoid the behavior and situations that lead to eating the wrong foods. Perhaps you need to temporarily stop having lunch at a fast-food restaurant with your coworkers. Perhaps you need to take a different route home so that you do not pass that pizzeria. Perhaps you need to stop eating in front of the television. You know best which are your food triggers. Once you identify them, combat them. You may find yourself having a lot of internal dialogue, as two sides of your brain argue with each other. However you do it, the object is to focus on the long term: a thinner, healthier, happier you.

Food, Glorious Low Carb Food

Now we'll move on to Part Three, where you will find delicious menus and recipes to help you enjoy all the amazing low carb foods you still have to discover. You've come a long way from where you were when you first picked up this book. You're eating delicious, formerly forbidden fare. You may be noticing with amazement that food doesn't rule your life anymore. You may even find that you sometimes forget to eat! You've rediscovered your energy and vitality, perhaps. Maybe you're sleeping better and feeling less moody and irritable. Is all of this worth giving up your old favorite junk foods? We know the answer, and now you do, too.

▶ Food for Thought

Your two weeks on Induction have been filled with changes. Take a look back on that period of time, then use your answers to the following questions to help you determine whether you should remain on Induction or move on to OWL.

When you think back over the last two weeks . . .

What has been easier than you expected?

_____
_____
_____

What did you find easier to do than on other programs?

_____
_____
_____

What was more difficult?

_____
_____
_____

Do you find yourself less preoccupied with food?

_____

_____

_____

Do you put less on your plate or find yourself satisfied
sooner?

_____

_____

_____

Are you coping better with all of your usual stresses?

_____

_____

_____

Do you wake with more energy?

_____

_____

_____

Do you have to push yourself less?

_____

_____

_____

What foods do you miss most?

_____

_____

_____

What foods did you think you would miss but did not actually miss?

_____

_____

_____

Do you believe that this is a way of eating you can make a lifestyle?

_____

_____

_____

What foods do you look forward to reintroducing into your meals?

_____

_____

_____

PART THREE

It's All About the Food

10 ► Eating In

I was a carbohydrate junkie so I desperately wanted bread for the first four days. I managed to get through the first two weeks of Induction, during which I lost 17 pounds. I had dropped a whole dress size! Soon, the cravings stopped altogether but to get through snack attacks, my strategy was to have a stock of fresh vegetables and macadamia nuts in the house at all times. Now I know that change is always possible—it's all a question of mindset. I feel reborn and have vowed to myself that I will never be fat again.

—Maehing Schenk, lost 86 pounds

At last! You've arrived at the part of the book that brings out the gastronomic gusto in all of us. It's time to put the things you've learned in the previous chapters into practice—and the delicious news is, that involves *eating*. We're no longer just talking about the rich-tasting, perhaps formerly "forbidden" foods you can enjoy on Atkins, we're about to dig into them.

How to do it? For most of us, there are two choices: cooking for ourselves, or getting our meals outside the home, whether we sit down at a restaurant or dash in for that carryout bag. Either way, it's important that you think ahead of time about what (and where) you'll be eating. In this chapter, we'll tackle the former, so tie on your apron and let's get started! (In Chapter 11, we'll provide dependable dining-out strategies.)

▶ Stocking Your Kitchen

To breeze through Induction, go shopping a day or two before you begin, and fill your fridge, freezer and pantry with foods from the "Acceptable Induction Foods" list in Chapter 5. When you have all you need right in the house, you will be less tempted to eat the wrong things or go out for fast food after a long day at the office.

REFRIGERATOR REQUISITES

- **Cheeses:** Keep on hand several types for snacks and to liven up salads. Buy small quantities to prevent waste.
- **Eggs:** Have a few hard-boiled eggs in the fridge at all times. They make the perfect protein snack as is, or can be made into deviled eggs.
- **Protein:** Purchase your meat, fish and poultry frequently to ensure freshness, and cook the

same day. If you freeze them, defrost in the refrigerator.

- **Tofu:** Also known as bean curd and made from soybeans, it is another good source of protein.
- **Cold cuts:** Baked ham, smoked turkey, corned beef and sliced roast beef are great for snacks and salad additions.
- **Salad vegetables:** Buy only five days' worth. Wash and wrap greens to preserve freshness and make quick work of salad preparation.
- **Vegetables:** Depending on the season, buy broccoli, green and yellow squash, cauliflower, eggplant, green beans, jicama, mushrooms, asparagus, bell peppers, green onions, leeks, spinach and broccoflower.

PANTRY PRACTICALITIES

- **Canned tuna:** The top pantry protein staple. For salads, tuna packed in water is milder and blends better with other ingredients. Tuna in oil (preferably olive oil) stands up well to cooked vegetables and stronger condiments, making it a better base for hot entrées.
- **Canned salmon and canned crabmeat:** These are excellent alternatives to tuna in salads; and salmon is higher in calcium than milk.
- **Sugar substitute:** In granular form, it can be used cup for cup for sugar in baking; packets are perfect for sweetening beverages.

- **Spices and dried herbs:** These can transform plain foods like grilled chicken into tasty ethnic specialties. Try basil to make it Italian, chili powder to make it Mexican and tarragon to make it French.
- **Low carb salad dressings and sauces:** Products like Atkins Quick Quisine™ Barbecue Sauce and Teriyaki Sauce dress up main dishes and vegetables in one quick pour.

FREEZER FUNDAMENTALS

- Spinach
- Kale
- Collards
- Snow peas
- Green beans
- Artichoke hearts
- Asparagus spears
- Chopped broccoli
- Unsweetened strawberries, blueberries, raspberries
- Rhubarb
- Frozen cooked shrimp
- Frozen crabmeat (real, not artificial)
- Low carb sliced bread

▶ Great Gadgets for Easy Low Carb Meals

In addition to the right foods, a few kitchen tools can make becoming a controlled carb cook a snap:

- **Instant-read thermometer.** Be sure protein sources such as beef, chicken and pork are cooked long enough to kill off microorganisms, but not so long that they get tough or dry.
- **Slow cooker.** When it comes to convenience, nothing beats a slow cooker. Leave for work in the morning and have a home-cooked meal when you arrive home. It's ideal for cooking less expensive cuts of meat, since they cook in their own juices all day.
- **Immersion blender.** This versatile, light hand-held blender goes right into a sauce or soup to blend ingredients.
- **Knife sharpener.** Sharp knives make chopping and slicing easier. Invest in a set of good quality knives, too.
- **Grill pan or indoor grill.** Get the taste of the outdoors all year long with a grill pan or a countertop grill. It's one of the fastest ways to cook chicken, fish or burgers.

Once the cabinets, fridge and freezer are stockpiled with those must-haves, you can whip up snacks and meals that are easy to grab when you're on the go.

➤ Wake Up to an Array of Breakfast Choices

Searching for breakfast foods that aren't sky-high in carbohydrates or nutrient deficient? It can seem like a tall order when you consider that a typical bowl of cereal—even one of the unsweetened so-called "healthy" brands—plus milk contains about 35 grams of carbohydrates. Doughnuts, toaster pastries, bagels, frozen waffles, and pancakes are, not surprisingly, sugary carb catastrophes; worse still, most contain dangerous trans fats.

Fortunately, there are low carb alternatives to the usual breakfast fare. The traditional favorite, eggs, may be too time-consuming for preparing omelets, frittatas and poached dishes every morning, but hard-boiled eggs can easily be made in advance and kept in the fridge. For accompaniments to eggs, snatch up precooked sausage patties, precooked bacon and similar high protein foods in the frozen foods section of your supermarket—they can be heated quickly in the microwave or toaster oven. Cheese slices, sliced tomatoes, avocado, even leftovers from the night before, are quick to prepare and satisfying. Try thinking outside conventional options, too, by experimenting with ideas for whitefish salad, tuna salad or chicken salad.

Thanks to Atkins Bakery™ Ready-to-Eat Sliced White, Whole-Grain or Rye Bread, with only 3 grams of Net Carbs per slice, you can enjoy toast with butter during Induction (stick to one slice). Other breakfast treats suitable for Induction include:

- Pancakes and waffles made with Atkins Quick Quisine™ Pancake & Waffle Mixes; drizzle them with Atkins Quick Quisine™ Sugar Free Pancake Syrup and melted butter.
- If you can't imagine starting the day without cereal, you'll be pleased to know there's also high fiber Atkins® Hot Cereal.
- For those frantic mornings when you just can't sit down to a real breakfast, take the grab-and-go approach with an Atkins Advantage™ Bar, an Atkins Morning Start™ Breakfast Bar or an Atkins Advantage™ Ready-to-Drink Shake.

THE PERFECT FOOD

Eggs are such a compact form of nutrition that they're often called the perfect food. One large egg provides 70 calories, 6 grams of protein, less than 1 gram of carbohydrate, 4.5 grams of fat and generous amounts of many vitamins and minerals. In fact, the only nutrient completely absent from the egg is vitamin C—chickens, unlike humans, manufacture all they need.

A large egg also contains 215 milligrams of cholesterol. But dietary cholesterol does not automatically become blood cholesterol when you eat it. The majority of the cholesterol in your blood is actually made by your own body. The quantity it

makes is determined by your weight and heredi-
tary factors. If you are controlling your carbohydrate intake by doing Atkins, the cholesterol in
eggs should pose no health risk.

Egg consumption is on the rise, and for good
reason. Research shows that high cholesterol
foods such as egg yolks are rarely responsible for
elevated levels of blood cholesterol. One study,
conducted by researchers at Michigan State University, showed that people who ate four or more
eggs per week actually had lower levels of blood
cholesterol than those who didn't eat eggs. The
egg eaters obtained more of all nutrients except vitamin B6 and fiber than those who didn't eat eggs
on a regular basis.

Egg yolks are an excellent source of nutrients.
They are one of the few foods that provide vitamin
D, and they boast respectable amounts of ri-
boflavin, folate, vitamin A and selenium. It makes
sense to eat such a potent source of nutrients
rather than just the egg whites or cholesterol-free
egg substitutes. These products are usually egg
whites that have been processed with coloring
agents (to mimic the yolk's color), natural flavors,
spices, vitamins and minerals (to replace those
from the lost yolk), an anti-greening agent and sta-
bilizers such as vegetable gums. Remember, as
long as you are keeping your carbohydrate intake
under control, you can eat healthy fats while lowering your total cholesterol.

► Lunch Done Right

You won't get the lunchtime doldrums if you get a little creative with that midday meal. After all, it can be
your much-needed chance to relax and refuel so you
can power through the rest of your afternoon. These
lunch picks will keep your motor running:

- **Chicken salad, tuna salad, or turkey salad.**
  Serve on a bed of lettuce with other fresh veggies or make an open-face sandwich with a
  slice of low carb bread.
- **Quick quesadillas.** Fill low carb tortillas with
  meats, vegetables and cheese and pan-fry or
  brush with oil and bake.
- **Wraps.** Stuff a low carb tortilla with avocado
  slices, chicken, sprouts and other veggies and
  sliced chicken or another protein.
- **Leftovers.** If you roast a chicken the night before, use the meat as a base for either a salad or
  an open-face sandwich.
- **Caesar salad, Cobb salad, chef salad.** Any
  salad that contains proteins (cheese, poultry,
  luncheon meat made without nitrates) and low
  carb dressing is a healthy option.
- **Omelets.** If you haven't had eggs for breakfast,
  a filled omelet loaded with vegetables makes a
  good lunch.
- **Burger.** Just hold the bun and serve with a side
  salad. Top with cheese if you wish.

- **Steak, lobster.** Dinner for lunch. Treat yourself. A juicy steak or a lobster tail with a side of veggies is a great way to beat lunchtime boredom.
- **Low carb soups in a cup.** They are warming and filling when paired with a hearty side salad.

AT THE READY

With these meal-makers in the fridge, there should be no "What can I eat?" crises:

- Grill and slice flank steak for a cold beef salad, a hearty snack, or for threading onto skewers (serve with low carb blue cheese dressing).
- Make chicken salad with boneless chicken breasts (buy them precooked to save time); or simply cut grilled chicken breasts into slices for topping salads or between-meal munching.
- Keep a bowl of tuna salad made with mayo and chopped celery in the fridge for quick lunches or a different breakfast option.
- Cut cheese cubes and divide into four 1-ounce portions to snack on, melt over chicken or steak or add to salads.
- Cut celery, cucumbers and zucchini sticks and keep them in a resealable plastic bag; use your favorite low carb salad dressing for dipping.
- Toss lettuce, cucumber, celery and/or other salad vegetables, divide into two-cup servings, and store in resealable plastic bags for superfast salads.

- Store hard-boiled eggs and crisp-cooked bacon in plastic containers for salad garnishes.
- Cook spaghetti squash and divide into one-cup servings (microwave with a couple of table-spoons of heavy cream, some grated Parmesan cheese, sage, salt and pepper).
- Chop and sauté collard, beet or dandelion greens with kale or chard and keep refriger-ated to add to hot bouillon broth.
- Wrap sliced roasted turkey and sliced cheese with a lettuce leaf.

► Dinnertime

Dinner is perhaps the easiest meal to make when you're doing Atkins. Start with your protein dish, whether poultry, fish or meat. You can broil it, bake it, sauté it or fry it (so long as you don't use flour or bread crumbs). Then add a small salad and a serving of cooked vegetables, and you're set to go. You can even have a sugar-free pudding or gelatin with whipped cream for dessert.

THE SKINNY ON FATTY FISH

In addition to being a great source of protein, fish is a rich source of many other nutrients, including a compound found in few other foods that is absolutely essential for your body to function. Fish vary considerably in flavor and texture, so if you don't enjoy one type, there are many others to try. Fish also vary in their nutritional makeup but, in general, all fish supply considerable amounts of protein, iron, the B vitamins and vitamins E, A and K. Perhaps most significantly, fatty fish is one of the few dietary sources of omega-3 fatty acids.

Omega-3s are a type of essential fatty acid—and essential means that the body requires it, but it cannot manufacture it. Omega-3s are found in canola oil, walnuts, soybeans, flaxseed oil and fish, but those that are found in fish are a special type that appear to protect against coronary artery disease.

Here are some popular fish and their grams of omega-3s (based on a 6-ounce cooked serving, except where noted):

- Atlantic salmon, farmed   3.7 g
- Atlantic salmon, wild   3.1 g
- Sardines in oil (3 ounces)   2.8 g
- Herring, kippered (3 ounces)   1.8 g
- Rainbow trout, wild   1.7 g
- Swordfish   1.4 g

Omega-3s are also found in mackerel, tuna, eel and cod.

11 ▶ Eating Out

Today, cooking three square meals at home can seem like an almost prehistoric concept. Crammed schedules with little time to spend in the kitchen, not to mention the extensive array of restaurant, takeout and prepared meal options, as well as diminishing emphasis on culinary skills through the generations, mean many of us rely on others to feed us. Indeed, according to the National Restaurant Association, almost half of all Americans eat at least one meal outside the home on a typical day. And a little more than one-fifth of us order takeout or delivery. These significant changes in how and where we eat are undoubtedly part of the reason for the nation's obesity crisis.

While preparing your own meals is the only sure way to know exactly what you're getting, you'd be hard-pressed to find a weight-loss program that's easier to follow when dining out than Atkins. No matter what kind of cuisine you crave, you'll have options that will keep you satisfied—and you'll never have to pass on a dinner invitation because "I'm trying to lose weight." Check out what you need to know to eat out while you slim down.

► **Distress-Free Dining Out**

Once you've understood the rules of Induction, you're primed with everything you need to navigate your favorite restaurant menu. Now, however, you'll be looking at the offerings in a different light, as you separate acceptable items—like a juicy cheddar burger sans bun, roast chicken with buttery sautéed asparagus, or stir-fried beef and broccoli—from those no-no's, such as pasta, rice and bread. Your newfound knowledge might even open your eyes to some palate-pleasers that you've never sampled before! Here, some helpful hints for dining out anywhere:

- **Don't show up ravenous.** When you skip a meal or arrive at the restaurant super-hungry, you may lose your self-control when you come face to face with the breadbasket or high carb appetizers. Instead, enjoy a hard-boiled egg, a few slices of cheese or even half an Atkins Advantage™ Bar before you go out. You can also ask for some steamed veggies to nibble on before your main course arrives.

- **Drink up.** A couple of glasses of water before your meal can help quell your appetite. Say no to diet sodas—the sugar substitutes used in most of them will only intensify your carb cravings.

- **Be adventurous.** Try one or two dishes you've never had before instead of ordering the same ones time after time. If you're bored with the foods you're eating, it's harder to stick to your weight-control regimen, so go for variety.

- **Check out the scene online**. Many restaurants feature their menus on the Internet. Try to visit the establishment's Web site to review the offerings and map out your dining plan ahead of time.

- **Forget the extras**. Ask your server to omit the rice, beans, potatoes or pasta. Most restaurants will also accommodate requests for a portion of vegetables in lieu of such high carb starches. (Thanks to the success of Atkins, you may even find a special low carb section on restaurant menus.)

- **Take sides**. Ask for sauces on the side so you can decide whether and how much to consume.

- **Start with soup**. It is an ideal way to curb your appetite. Miso soup, many cream soups and clear broth with meat or vegetables are all satisfying and delicious ways to jump-start a controlled carb meal.

- **Never save room for dessert**. Go ahead and fill up on everything else so that you are satiated by the end of the meal and not prone to temptation.

- **Don't go there**. Don't give in to an "I deserve it" mentality. What you deserve is to be healthy while still enjoying the foods you already love, not succumbing to unhealthy indulgences.

- **Accept an occasional misstep**. Don't torture yourself if you accidentally consume something that's been batter-dipped or breaded. Remember that it's only one meal.

- **Be a copycat**. If there's a low carb dish you particularly relish at a restaurant, ask if you can find out how to make it at home. That way you can add to your repertoire of favorites and enjoy it as often as you like!

▶ Low Carb Globetrotting

From the biggest cities to small-town USA, wherever you live, the experience of dining out can take you on an intercontinental journey. Whether you favor French fare or you're partial to pizza, there are foods to choose and foods to avoid.

AT THAI RESTAURANTS . . .

Influenced by the cuisine of neighboring Indonesia and China, Thai food is largely rice- and noodle-based. But there are still plenty of options when you're doing Atkins, including a large variety of fish and shellfish dishes. In general, Thai food is light and contains heady combinations of herbs and spices to yield sour, salty, hot and sweet flavors. Avoid deep-fried dishes and stick to those that are quickly sautéed with lemon-grass and/or basil, as well as other aromatic Thai herbs and vegetables.

Choose:
- *Tom yum koong*: shrimp and mushrooms sim-mered in hot-and-sour broth with coriander, lime leaves and lemongrass
- Sautéed shrimp or beef with basil, onion and chilies
- Sautéed scallops and shrimp (or beef or pork) with mushrooms, zucchini and chili paste
- Sautéed beef, chicken or pork or sautéed veg-etables
- Steamed mussels with Thai herbs and garlic sauce

Avoid:
- Dumplings or spring rolls
- Bean thread, a vermicelli-like noodle
- Pad Thai and anything else listed as *pad*; it will almost certainly be a noodle dish.
- Curry dishes that contain potatoes
- Dishes that use sweet ingredients, such as pineapple, oyster sauce, and sweet-and-sour sauce
- Dishes with black bean sauce
- Thai fried rice
- Deep-fried whole fish with sweet-and-sour sauce

AT ITALIAN RESTAURANTS . . .

At first glance, eating at an Italian restaurant might seem impossible, as you would have to bypass pastas, bean dishes and risottos. However, a delicious variety of traditional recipes can still be savored. Look to grilled specialties from wood-burning ovens that are used for preparing more than just pizza. And zero in on chicken, veal, fish or shrimp (scampi) sautéed in butter or olive oil and garlic or roasted to perfection.

Choose:
- Salads tossed with olive oil and vinegar; avoid balsamic vinegar, which is high in sugar
- *Insalata Caprese*: sliced tomatoes, mozzarella cheese and fresh basil drizzled with olive oil
- *Antipasto:* assorted meats and cheeses, marinated peppers and mushrooms, and clams
- *Prosciutto:* air-cured ham with a delicate, slightly salty flavor, usually sliced paper-thin and served with slices of melon or layered with veal scallops (skip the melon)
- Steamed or buttery mussels or clams
- A cup of clear broth, or *stracciatella*, Italian egg-drop soup—make sure it contains no pasta or beans
- Shrimp, steamed or in garlic butter
- Sautéed, grilled or marinated *calamari* or *scungilli* (squid or octopus)
- Broccoli rabe or the vegetable of the day, drizzled with a touch of olive oil and garlic, if you choose

- Simply prepared chicken, fish and meat offerings that have been grilled, broiled or poached in oil, butter or broth.
- *Piccata* or *saltimbocca* (layered with prosciutto and spinach) dishes, which are not prepared in a batter
- Grilled fish, chicken, beef or veal
- Marsala dishes, which are cooked in wine

Avoid:
- Breaded starters, like fried mozzarella and *calamari fritti*, and garlic bread
- Shrimp cocktail—the sauce may be full of sugar
- Veal dishes such as *Franchese* or *Parmesan,* which are breaded before frying
- Lasagna, noodle and pasta dishes
- Dishes with tomato sauce; carb counts can vary widely. Request sauce made from chopped, fresh tomatoes

AT FRENCH RESTAURANTS . . .

The traditional French diet includes fish, meats and vegetables cooked with full-fat cheeses, butter and rich sauces, most of which are yours to enjoy on Induction. Watch out for breads and bean dishes.

Choose:
- Pâté, made from liver
- Escargots (snails), which are typically cooked in butter

- Foie gras, fattened duck liver
- Consommé, clear broth
- *Soupe à l'oignon*: onion soup; ask to have it prepared without the bread
- Meat, fish or chicken that's baked, broiled or roasted without flour-thickened sauces or cooked in a simple sauté of butter or oil
- Filet mignon
- *Salad Nicoise*: lettuce, hard-boiled egg, potatoes, string beans, anchovies; remove the potato and request oil-and-vinegar dressing
- *Coquilles Saint-Jacques*: scallops in wine sauce
- *Coq au vin*: chicken simmered in wine sauce; remove any potatoes or carrots
- *Navarin d'agneau*: leg of lamb, usually larded with slivers of garlic and rubbed with fragrant olive oil and fresh rosemary before roasting or grilling
- *Steak-frite*: steak with french fries; ask your server to hold the "*frites*," and replace with a side of low carb vegetables
- Lamb or duck dishes without flour-based sauces, or *roux*
- Dishes made with béarnaise sauce, which is made from egg yolks and butter
- *Ratatouille*: a Provençal casserole of eggplant, tomatoes, onions, peppers and zucchini; the vegetables are sometimes dredged in flour before cooking, so check with your server before ordering it as a side dish

Avoid:

- *Caneton à l'orange*: whole roast duck served in a sweetened sauce, flavored with orange juice and orange sections. A similar dish made with prunes (*au pruneaux*) or cherries (*aux cerises*) is also off-limits during Induction

- *Cassoulet*: a casserole made largely of white beans, along with preserved duck, pork loin, bacon, lamb and garlic sausage

- *Bouef bourguignon*: cubes of beef dredged in flow, then simmered in red wine with beef broth, garlic, tiny onions and herbs

At Greek and Middle Eastern Restaurants . . .

It's hard to make too many missteps when you sit down to a Greek or Middle Eastern meal—almost all entrées are charcoal-grilled, wood-grilled or broiled. Olive oil, lemon, garlic and onions are central ingredients in Mediterranean cuisine, as are eggplant, okra, lemon, cauliflower and green beans. Lamb is the preferred protein, and whether stewed, roasted, pressed, ground or skewered, it dominates the menu. Mint tea will fill you up and aid digestion. Although the yogurt served in Greek restaurants is usually the full-fat kind, which is lower in carbs than low fat versions, pass on it until you are beyond Induction.

Choose:

- Kebobs: skewered meats, chicken or fish, which are often seasoned with spices and served with grilled or roasted vegetables

- Kofta, which are balls of ground lamb and onions that are skewered and grilled
- Greek salad, loaded with fresh greens, peppers and tomatoes and topped with feta cheese, olives, oil and lemon. Remove the grape leaves stuffed with rice.
- Souvlaki, marinated and thin-sliced meat; remove pita-bread wrapping
- Eggplant, often cooked with garlic, tomatoes and peppers
- Baba ghanoush, a spread similar to hummus, but made with eggplant instead of chickpeas

Avoid:
- Gyros: pita sandwiches stuffed with ground beef or lamb; pita bread can have 50 or more grams of carbs
- *Spanakopita*: spinach pie, which is made with phyllo dough, which ups the carb content
- *Dolmades*: grape leaves, which are often stuffed with rice in addition to ground lamb
- *Moussaka*: a popular Greek eggplant casserole of lamb, eggplant and cheese held together with a béchamel sauce made with bleached flour
- *Tzatziki*, or "yogurt sauce"
- Hummus: a dip made from chickpeas, garlic and sesame paste
- *Kibbe*: patties made of ground lamb and bulgur
- *Tabbouleh*: bulgur (cracked wheat) salad
- *Fattoush*, a bread, cucumber and tomato salad
- *Falafel*: fried patties made from mashed chickpeas and spices

At Japanese and Sushi Restaurants . . .

Raw fish and vegetables are the focal point, although chicken and beef usually make an appearance on the menu. Steer clear of the sticky rice and seek out some of the exciting Japanese flavors in the form of *shoyu* (soy sauce), *mirin* (rice wine), *dashi* (a flavorful broth made from dried bonito fish flakes), *ponzu* (a dipping sauce made from soy sauce, rice-wine vinegar, dashi and seaweed), *wasabi* (extra-pungent horseradish), pickled ginger, miso (soybean paste) and sesame seeds and sesame oil.

Choose:
- Seaweed salad
- Miso soup
- *Ebi-su* (shrimp)
- *Yakitori* (skewered chicken and onions broiled in teriyaki sauce and served on a skewer)
- *Oshinko* (pickled cabbage)
- *Ohitashi* (boiled spinach with sesame seeds)
- *Shabu-shabu*: thin slices of beef, quickly cooked with mushrooms, cabbage and other vegetables
- Broiled dishes, often referred to as *yakimono*
- *Sashimi*: sliced raw fish, served with wasabi (Japanese horseradish), soy sauce and pickled ginger

Avoid:
- Vegetable dishes prepared tempura-style
- Deep-fried dumplings
- Sushi, which combines raw fish with rice rolled in sheets of *nori*, or seaweed
- Noodle soups or dishes

AT KOREAN RESTAURANTS . . .

Korean cuisine benefits from a merging of Mongolian, Japanese and Chinese culinary traditions. Menus offer a wide array of beef dishes and spicy options. A typical meal might include a bowl of soup followed by a grilled or stir-fried main course, plus several small plates (as many as 10 or more) called *panchan*, containing sauces, pickles, preserved fish and other condiments. Ask your server to leave the rice bowl in the kitchen.

Choose:
- *Bulgogi* (sometimes spelled *pulgogi* or *bul go gui*): Korean barbecue, or thin slices of beef (either rib eye, sirloin or prime rib) steeped in a fragrant barbecue sauce and cooked over a charcoal grill at your table
- *Kal bi tang* (sometimes spelled *galbi tang*): marinated beef-rib stew, sometimes served off the bone
- *Kimchi*: hot-and-spicy vegetable nibbles
- Cold or fried tofu
- *Twoenjang guk:* fermented soybean-paste soup with baby clams

- Seafood soup
- *Shinsollo:* meat, fish, vegetables and tofu simmered in beef broth
- *Ny go gi:* barbecued beef, chicken, pork or fish

Avoid:

- *Pa jon*: a scallion pancake made of rice flour and egg and pieces of beef or shrimp; served with a soy-sauce–based dip
- *Mandoo guk*: beef stew served with Korean dumplings, similar to Chinese wontons
- *Bimibap* (sometimes spelled *pibimpap* or *-bop*): a rice-based casserole (*bap/bop* means rice) mixed with pieces of meat, seasoned vegetables and egg
- *Myon noodle dishes*: buckwheat noodles in broth with a variety of other ingredients such as beef, shredded radishes and cucumbers
- *Chapchae*: transparent rice noodles, along with beef, mushrooms, green onions and vegetables with sesame oil

At Fast-Food Restaurants . . .

They dot the landscape from coast to coast, and their ready-to-go selections and reasonable prices can make them hard to resist. Aim to limit your visits to these ubiquitous establishments. Make the smartest choices possible when you do find yourself at the drive-thru.

Quick Tips:
- Think small. Don't super-size it, no matter how good the deal.
- Ask for bottled water instead of soda.
- At salad bars, avoid the croutons as well as bean, pasta and potato salads.
- Check out the nutrition information, which is typically posted on the wall near the counter, or ask for a nutrition brochure.

AT BURGER CHAINS . . .

All of the sandwiches, from cheeseburgers to grilled-chicken sandwiches, can typically be transformed into an Atkins-friendly choice simply by tossing the bun. Avoid breaded fish or chicken dishes. Mayonnaise and mustard are permissible but forgo the ketchup packets, which contain added sugar. Skip special sauces, which may also contain sugar. Pile on lettuce and tomato for garnish. Many burger chains now offer salads and grilled items—good options if you choose sugar-free salad dressing.

AT SALAD BARS . . .

Start with a base of lettuce and acceptable vegetables, then top with protein foods such as hard-boiled eggs, turkey or chicken. Avoid coleslaw, which may contain sugar, and pasta salads. Use oil and regular red- or white-wine vinegar instead of a prepared dressing; commercial dressings and balsamic vinegars often contain sugar. Also pass on the baked stuffed potatoes.

At Fried-Chicken Joints . . .

Barbecue sauce is full of sugar, and even if you remove the skin from the chicken, the sugar has probably seeped into the meat. Dry-rubbed meats, roasted chicken and acceptable side dishes such as salad are good picks. Discard the bun on the grilled-chicken sandwich, and, if necessary, scrape breading off fried chicken breasts.

At Pizza Parlors . . .

The options won't be extensive here. Most pizza parlors offer a salad. Top with luncheon meats, if available. If absolutely necessary, order a pizza and eat only the cheese and toppings. It's messy, but you'll avoid the high carb crust.

At Mexican-Style Restaurants . . .

Chicken or beef tacos with lettuce, cheese and grilled chicken will do, as long as you unload the shells and eat the remaining ingredients with a fork as a "salad." Steer clear of combination plates loaded with rice and beans.

At Sandwich and Sub Shops . . .

Chicken or tuna salad is a smart choice, as are turkey, roast beef and cheese. Avoid salami, bologna and other meat products preserved with nitrates. Simply ask for your selection on a plate instead of on a roll.

12 ► Two Weeks of Delicious Eating and Recipes for Induction

Food is one of life's greatest pleasures. These meal plans and recipes help prove it by incorporating the most appealing flavors and ingredients while they make adhering to the Atkins Nutritional Approach™ worry-free and easy.

► It's All About the Food

To help guide you through two weeks of Induction, we've created 14 daily meal plans, each tallying no more than 20 grams of Net Carbs distributed throughout the day. You'll find loads of variety to keep your taste buds tantalized. Breakfasts include eggs, cereal, pancakes and waffles; lunches feature main dish salads, a variety of burgers and open-face sandwiches; and dinner selections offer up well-seasoned protein, more salads and nutritionally dense vegetables. We haven't forgotten sweets and snacks, either!

One note: **Be sure to heed the given amounts for salad dressings and sauces, since these items contain carbs. When it comes to vinegar, remember to stick with red wine, cider and white vinegars, since most balsamic contains added sugar.** (To order Atkins brand and other low carb products mentioned in the meal plans, visit *www.atkins.com.*)

If you're short on time, take heart: you can whip up most of the recipes in less than 30 minutes, while your kitchen fills with exhilarating aromas that can come only from home-cooking. There's something to please every palate, too. Whether you sink your teeth into a juicy Cheddar Burger with Cherry Pepper Sauce, try out Olé Turkey Tacos or give fish a whirl in Halibut with Herbed Brown Butter, you'll find dishes that meet the expectations of your taste buds without compromising your weight-loss goals. Chocolate Mudslide and Vanilla Flan are the sweet endings that round out your meals and keep you focused on losing pounds and feeling your best. Happy eating!

Note: Recipes for asterisked meal plan items can be found in the recipe section (see pages 207–230).

▶ ◀

Two-Week Meal Plan
for Induction

DAY 1

Breakfast

2 eggs, scrambled	1
3 slices Canadian bacon	1
1 slice Atkins Bakery™ Ready-to-Eat Sliced Multigrain Bread	3
	5

Lunch

Shrimp salad	0
1 cup spinach salad with olive oil and vinegar	2
1 small tomato, sliced	4
	6

Dinner

*Spiced Lamb Chop**	1
½ cup sautéed Swiss chard with 1 tablespoon lemon juice	2
1 cup mixed greens with 2 tablespoons Atkins™ Sweet French Dressing	2
	5

Snack

5 large black olives and 2 ounces cheese	3
	3

TOTAL GRAMS NET CARBS: 19

DAY 2

Breakfast
Smoked salmon, cucumber and cream
cheese roll-ups   1
1 small tomato, sliced   4
                                                      ———
                                                         5

Lunch
*Cheddar Burger with
Cherry Pepper Sauce**   1
2 cups mesclun with oil and vinegar   4
                                                      ———
                                                         5

Dinner
Roast chicken   0
½ cup broccoli with Parmesan cheese curls   3
⅔ cup endive and radish salad with
2 tablespoons Atkins™ Sweet
Poppyseed Dressing   2
                                                      ———
                                                         5

Snack
½ cup red pepper strips with blue cheese
dressing (combine 2 tablespoons
crumbled blue cheese, mayonnaise and
sour cream, to taste)   4.5
                                                      ———
                                                       4.5

TOTAL GRAMS NET CARBS: 19.5

DAY 3

Breakfast

½ cup Atkins® Hot Cereal	3
1 hard-boiled egg	0.5
	3.5

Lunch

Cobb salad: grilled chicken, ½ diced tomato, bacon, ½ avocado, and 2 tablespoons crumbled blue cheese over 1 cup greens with oil and vinegar	5.5
	5.5

Dinner

Grilled salmon with 2 tablespoons Atkins Quick Quisine™ Teriyaki Sauce	2
*Sesame Green Beans**	5
Cabbage slaw: ½ cup shredded cabbage, mayonnaise and celery seed, to taste	1
	8

Snack

Atkins Advantage™ Chocolate Peanut Butter Bar	2
	2

TOTAL GRAMS NET CARBS: **19**

DAY 4

Breakfast

Greek omelet: ½ cup spinach, 2 ounces
feta and 2 eggs   5
                                                                 —
                                                                 5

Lunch

Open-face Reuben: corned beef, 2 slices
Swiss cheese, ¼ cup sauerkraut and
1 slice Atkins Bakery™
Ready-to-Eat Sliced Rye Bread   6
                                                                 —
                                                                 6

Dinner

Grilled sirloin steak   0
*Asparagus with Tarragon Vinaigrette**   4
1 cup mixed green salad with blue
cheese dressing (combine 2 tablespoons
crumbled blue cheese, mayonnaise
and sour cream, to taste)   2
                                                                 —
                                                                 6

Snack

1 celery stalk with 2 tablespoons soy
nut butter   2
                                                                 —
                                                                 2

TOTAL GRAMS NET CARBS: 19

DAY 5

Breakfast

3 pancakes made from Atkins Quick Quisine™ Pancake & Waffle Mix	3
1 tablespoon Atkins Quick Quisine™ Sugar Free Pancake Syrup	0
3 turkey sausages	1
	4

Lunch

Tuna salad mixed with 1 stalk celery, 5 radishes and cherry tomato, all chopped	4
1 cup green salad with 2 tablespoons Atkins™ Sweet French Dressing	2
	6

Dinner

Roast pork tenderloin	0
1 cup sautéed spinach and red pepper with garlic	4
*Vanilla Flan**	2.5
	6.5

Snack

2 slices ham and 1 slice Swiss cheese wrapped around 1 dill pickle spear	3
	3

TOTAL GRAMS NET CARBS: 19.5

DAY 6

Breakfast

*Chicken and Egg Salad**	4.5
½ cup cucumber slices	1
	5.5

Lunch

Steak fajita: steak slices, one slice Monterey Jack cheese and a low carb tortilla	4
1 cup romaine hearts with olive oil and vinegar	4
	8

Dinner

Grilled tuna with spice rub	0
½ cup zucchini and ½ cup mushrooms grilled on skewers	2
1 cup arugula and endive salad with 1 tablespoon Atkins™ "Sweet as Honey" Mustard Dressing	3
	5

Snack

½ cup broccoli florets with lemon mayonnaise (combine 1 tablespoon lemon juice with mayonnaise)	1
	1

TOTAL GRAMS NET CARBS: 19.5

DAY 7

Breakfast

Poached egg on 1 slice Atkins Bakery™ Ready-to-Eat Sliced White Bread	3.5
1 slice beefsteak tomato	1
1 ounce Muenster cheese	0.5
	5

Lunch

Chef salad: thinly sliced ham, turkey, roast beef and chopped hard-boiled egg over 1 cup lettuce with olive oil and vinegar	2
	2

Dinner

Mushroom-Flavored Meatloaf*	3
⅓ cup each green beans, snow peas and bell pepper medley	6
1 cup green salad with olive oil and vinegar	2
	11

Snack

1 Atkins Quick Quisine™ Banana Nut Muffin	2
	2

TOTAL GRAMS NET CARBS: 　20

DAY 8

Breakfast

Atkins Morning Start™ Creamy	
Cinnamon Bun Breakfast Bar	2
2 pieces of string-cheese mozzarella	1.5
	3.5

Lunch

Chicken salad over 2 cups chopped	
red onion, jicama and mixed greens	5
1 low carb tortilla	3
	8

Dinner

Halibut with Herbed Brown Butter*	0
1 cup eggplant, pepper and tomato sauté	4.5
½ cup low carb vanilla pudding	1
	5.5

Snack

Shrimp cocktail (combine Atkins Quick	
Quisine™ Ketch-a-Tomato and jarred	
white horseradish for sauce)	3
	3

TOTAL GRAMS NET CARBS: **20**

DAY 9

Breakfast

*Zucchini and Swiss Cheese Frittata**   3
1 slice Atkins Bakery™
   Ready-to-Eat Sliced White Bread   3
                                            6

Lunch

½ avocado filled with crab salad (combine
   canned or frozen crab with mayo)   2
1 small tomato, sliced   4
2 cups baby lettuce with olive oil and
   vinegar   4
                                            10

Dinner

Roast beef au jus   0
1 cup roasted zucchini and mushrooms
   with herbs   2
Sugar-free gelatin   0
                                            2

Snack

Atkins Advantage™ Ready-to-Drink
   Chocolate Delight Shake   1
                                            1

TOTAL GRAMS NET CARBS: 19

DAY 10

Breakfast

Veggie wrap: 2 ounces Monterey Jack
cheese, 4 asparagus spears and 1 low
carb tortilla   6
                                              ———
                                                 6

Lunch

Sliced chicken breast   0
Tomato, Cucumber and Feta Salad*   5
                                              ———
                                                 5

Dinner

Baked ham steak drizzled with
1 tablespoon Atkins Quick Quisine™
Sugar Free Pancake Syrup   0
⅔ cup green beans tossed with chopped
mint   5
1 cup green salad with 2 tablespoons
Atkins™ Sweet Poppyseed Dressing   2
                                              ———
                                                 7

Snack

1 ounce cheese and 10 green olives   2
                                              ———
                                                 2

TOTAL GRAMS NET CARBS: 20

DAY 11

Breakfast

Atkins Morning Start™ Blueberry Muffin Breakfast Bar	2
1 soft-boiled egg	0.5
	2.5

Lunch

2 cups spinach salad with bacon and low carb blue cheese dressing (combine 2 tablespoons crumbled blue cheese, mayonnaise and sour cream, to taste)	3
1 slice Atkins Bakery™ Ready-to-Eat Sliced Multigrain Bread	3
	6

Dinner

Grilled Asian Pork Patties with Dipping Sauce*	3
1 cup red pepper, snow pea and green onion stir-fry	5
½ cup Chinese cabbage with sugar-free rice wine vinegar and sesame oil	2
	10

Snack

½ cup low carb chocolate pudding	1
	1

TOTAL GRAMS NET CARBS: 19.5

DAY 12

Breakfast

3 waffles made from Atkins Quick Quisine™ Pancake & Waffle Mix	3
1 tablespoon Atkins Quick Quisine™ Sugar Free Pancake Syrup	0
	3

Lunch

Turkey cheeseburger with 2 ounces Pepper Jack cheese	2
1 cup diced peppers, tomatoes and cucumber with oil and vinegar	5
	7

Dinner

Grilled veal chops with sage butter	0
⅔ cup sautéed yellow squash and ⅓ cup cherry tomatoes	4
1 cup green salad with olive oil and vinegar	2
	6

Snack

*Chocolate Mudslide**	2.5
	2.5

TOTAL GRAMS NET CARBS: 18.5

DAY 13

Breakfast

1 low carb tortilla filled with 2 eggs,
scrambled   4

1 tablespoon each green salsa and
sour cream   1
                                               ___
                                                5

Lunch

Open-face roast beef sandwich: roast beef,
1 slice Atkins Bakery™ Ready-to-
Eat Sliced Rye Bread and horseradish
mayonnaise (combine mayonnaise and
horseradish)   4

1 cup radish and cucumber salad with oil
and vinegar   2
                                               ___
                                                6

Dinner

Chicken with Tomato-Cream Sauce*   1.5
4 asparagus spears   2.5
1 cup mixed green salad with olive oil
and 1 tablespoon lemon juice   2
                                               ___
                                                6

Snack

Portobello-mushroom pizza (broiled
Portobello mushroom topped with
melted mozzarella cheese)   2
                                               ___
                                                2

TOTAL GRAMS NET CARBS: 19

DAY 14

Breakfast

Atkins Advantage™ Ready-to-Drink
Creamy Vanilla Shake   1
                                            ───
                                              1

Lunch

Olé Turkey Taco*   5
½ cup diced jicama salad with cilantro
and mayonnaise   3
                                            ───
                                              8

Dinner

Marinated grilled skirt steak   0
⅔ cup turnip fries with Atkins Quick
Quisine™ Ketch-a-Tomato Sauce   4
1 cup mixed green salad with low carb
blue cheese dressing (combine
2 tablespoons crumbled blue cheese,
mayonnaise and sour cream, to taste)   2
                                            ───
                                              6

Snack

1 small tomato stuffed
with egg salad   5
                                            ───
                                              5

TOTAL GRAMS NET CARBS: 20

Recipes for Induction

► Chicken with Tomato-Cream Sauce

You may use either dry- or oil-packed sun-dried tomatoes in this sauce. If using dry, add a tablespoon more broth and cook a little longer to allow the tomatoes to soften.

Prep time: 10 minutes
Cook time: 8 minutes
4 servings

4 boneless, skinless chicken breast halves (about 6 ounces each)
½ teaspoon salt
½ teaspoon chili powder
¼ teaspoon ground pepper
2 teaspoons olive oil
2 teaspoons butter
¼ cup chicken broth or water
2 tablespoons oil-packed dried tomatoes (about 6), cut into thin strips
½ cup heavy cream

1. Season chicken with salt, chili powder and pepper. In large skillet over medium-high heat melt butter in oil. Cook chicken 8 minutes, turning once, until cooked through. Remove to serving plate and keep warm.

2. Pour broth and tomatoes into pan and cook, stirring until liquid is reduced by half. Add cream, cook 4 minutes more until slightly thickened. Pour over chicken and serve immediately.

Per serving: carbohydrates: 2 grams; Net Carbs: 1.5 grams; fiber: 0.5 grams; protein: 40.5 grams; fat: 18 grams; calories: 338

▶ Halibut with Herbed Brown Butter

A flavorful butter sauce flecked with herbs enlivens mild-tasting fish such as halibut. If you prefer, substitute scrod or catfish fillets.

Prep time: 10 minutes
Cook time: 9 minutes
4 servings

2 tablespoons olive oil
4 halibut steaks, about 1 inch thick (6 to 8 ounces each)
¾ teaspoon salt, divided
¼ teaspoon ground pepper, divided
4 tablespoons butter
2 tablespoons mixed chopped fresh herbs, such as parsley, tarragon, basil and thyme
½ teaspoon fresh grated lemon rind

1. In large nonstick skillet, heat olive oil over high heat until it shimmers. Season fish with half the salt and pepper. Cook halibut 5 to 6 minutes, turning once, until just cooked through. Remove to serving plate; tent with foil to keep warm.

2. In same skillet, melt butter over medium-high heat. Cook about 3 minutes, until it bubbles and turns light brown. Remove from heat and add mixed herbs,

lemon rind and remaining salt and pepper. Pour sauce over fish and serve immediately.

Per serving: carbohydrates: 0 grams; Net Carbs: 0 grams; fiber: 0 grams; protein: 41.5 grams; fat: 23 grams; calories: 280

▶ Tomato, Cucumber and Feta Salad

Use the scale in the produce section to buy the appro-
priate amounts of tomatoes and cucumbers. We don't
use any olive oil in this recipe because the olives and
cheese add richness, but feel free to add some, to taste.

Prep time: 15 minutes
6 servings

1 pound tomatoes, seeded and cut into ½-inch pieces
1 pound cucumbers, seeded and cut into ½-inch pieces
1 teaspoon grated lemon rind
½ teaspoon salt
¼ teaspoon ground pepper
½ cup feta cheese, crumbled
½ cup cured black olives, pitted and chopped

1. In large salad bowl, toss tomatoes, cucumbers, lemon rind, salt and pepper. Let sit 15 minutes.
2. Top with feta and olives.

Per serving: carbohydrates: 7 grams; Net Carbs: 5
grams; fiber: 2 grams; protein: 3 grams; fat: 4 grams;
calories: 72

➤ Asparagus with Tarragon Vinaigrette

Asparagus is such an elegant vegetable it needs only a tangy vinaigrette to bring out its flavor.

Prep time: 10 minutes
Cook time: 10 minutes
4 servings

1 pound fresh asparagus, trimmed
2 tablespoons finely chopped red onion
2 tablespoons tarragon vinegar
1 teaspoon Dijon mustard
½ packet sugar substitute
½ teaspoon salt
¼ teaspoon ground pepper
¼ cup olive oil

1. Cook asparagus until crisp-tender. Drain, and pat dry with paper towels. Set aside.

2. Combine red onion, vinegar, mustard and sugar substitute, salt and pepper in a mixing bowl. Gradually whisk in oil. Pour dressing over asparagus, toss gently to coat.

Per serving: carbohydrates: 6 grams; Net Carbs: 4 grams; fiber: 2 grams; protein: 3 grams; fat: 14 grams; calories: 152

▶ Sesame Green Beans

Black sesame seeds can be found in some grocery stores and at Asian food markets. If you can't find them, toast regular sesame seeds in a skillet until they become fragrant.

Prep time: 15 minutes
Cook time: 7 minutes
Marinating time: 20 minutes
6 servings

1½ pounds green beans
3 tablespoons rice-wine vinegar
3 tablespoons low-sodium soy sauce
2 tablespoons black sesame seeds
1 teaspoon toasted sesame oil

1. In large pot of boiling salted water cook green beans about 7 minutes until crisp tender. Drain beans in a colander and transfer to a large zip-lock plastic bag or bowl. Toss beans with vinegar, soy sauce and sesame seeds until evenly coated. Let marinate 20 minutes, turning occasionally.

2. Drain marinade and toss beans with sesame oil. Serve at room temperature.

Per serving: carbohydrates: 9 grams; Net Carbs: 5 grams; fiber: 4 grams; protein: 2.5 grams; fat: 2.5 grams; calories: 62

▶ Spiced Lamb Chops

In this recipe we sear the lamb steaks first for a deep brown crust and then finish cooking them in the oven for a tender texture. However, if you like, you may finish the cooking right in the skillet.

Prep time: 5 minutes
Cook time: 10 minutes
4 servings

2 tablespoons curry powder
1 teaspoon salt
½ teaspoon freshly ground pepper
¼ teaspoon five-spice powder
1 tablespoon canola oil
4 leg of lamb steaks, ½ inch thick (about ¾ pound each)

1. Heat oven to 350°F. Combine curry, salt, pepper and five-spice powder in a cup. Sprinkle each side of steaks with 1 teaspoon of the spice mixture.

2. Heat oil in large skillet over medium-high heat; add 2 steaks and cook 1½ minutes per side just until deep brown. Transfer to broiler pan. Repeat browning process with the remaining 2 steaks.

3. Broil steaks 3 to 4 minutes until just pink in center or to desired doneness.

Per serving: carbohydrates: 2 grams; Net Carbs: 1 gram; fiber: 1 gram; protein: 60.5 grams; fat: 34 grams; calories: 556

▶ Cheddar Burgers with Cherry Pepper Sauce

In this recipe, we turned simple mayonnaise into a jazzy sauce by adding chopped cherry peppers and a dash of Worcestershire sauce.

Prep time: 10 minutes
Cook time: 10 minutes
4 servings

2 pounds ground beef chuck
4 teaspoons Atkins Quick Quisine™ Steak Sauce
½ teaspoon salt
1 cup (4 ounces) shredded cheddar cheese
¼ cup mayonnaise
1 small cherry pepper, drained and finely chopped
½ teaspoon Worcestershire sauce

1. Prepare a medium grill or heat broiler. Combine ground beef, steak sauce and salt. Form into 6 patties, about 3½ inches across by 1 inch thick.

2. Grill patties, covered, 5 minutes per side for medium-rare doneness (cook longer, if desired). Two minutes before the burgers are done top with cheddar cheese and cover grill.

3. While burgers are cooking, mix mayonnaise, cherry pepper and Worcestershire. Top burgers with sauce and serve.

Per serving: carbohydrates: 1 gram; Net Carbs: 1 gram; fiber: 0 grams; protein: 42.5 grams; fat: 39.5 grams; calories: 540

▶ Grilled Asian Pork Patties with Dipping Sauce

Pork patties are a welcome change of pace, and these are both tender and flavorful. Teriyaki sauce is the perfect complement to their subtle flavor.

Prep time: 15 minutes
Cook time: 12 minutes
6 servings

Patties:

2 pounds ground pork
¼ cup Atkins Quick Quisine™ Teriyaki Sauce
¼ cup green onions, white and green parts chopped
1 tablespoon chopped ginger
2 teaspoons chopped garlic

Sauce:

¼ cup Atkins Quick Quisine™ Teriyaki Sauce
1 tablespoon chopped green onion, white and green parts
2 teaspoons toasted sesame oil
1 teaspoon chopped ginger
1 teaspoon chopped garlic

1. **For patties:** Prepare a medium grill or heat broiler. Combine ground pork, teriyaki sauce, green onions, ginger and garlic. Form into 6 patties, a little less than ½ inch thick.

2. **For sauce:** Combine teriyaki sauce, green onion, sesame oil, ginger and garlic.

3. Grill patties 6 to 7 minutes per side until just cooked through. Serve with sauce.

Per serving: carbohydrates: 3 grams; Net Carbs: 3 grams; fiber: 0 grams; protein: 33.5 grams; fat: 30 grams; calories: 420

► Mushroom-Flavored Meatloaf

Mushrooms add moistness and flavor to this savory loaf. Leftover meatloaf makes great sandwiches, too, so plan ahead!

Prep time: 10 minutes
Cook time: 10 minutes
Bake time: 60 minutes
6 servings

2 slices Atkins Bakery™ Ready-to-Eat Sliced White Bread
1 tablespoon olive oil
2 cups sliced button mushrooms
1 teaspoon salt
1 large clove garlic
1½ pounds ground beef
½ of 1 medium onion, grated or minced
1 large egg
2 tablespoons spicy brown mustard
½ teaspoon freshly ground pepper

1. Heat oven to 350°F. Line a broiler pan bottom or baking sheet with foil or parchment. Pulse bread in a food processor until crumbs form, set aside.

2. Heat oil in 12-inch skillet over high heat. Add mushrooms; cook 8 to 9 minutes stirring once or twice until well browned. Sprinkle with salt and add garlic,

cook 30 to 60 seconds more until aromatic. Chop by hand or in food processor until very finely minced.

3. In a large bowl, gently combine meat with mushrooms and remaining ingredients until mixed. Form a 9" × 4" loaf on prepared pan; cover with foil and bake 30 minutes. Uncover and bake 30 to 35 minutes more until browned and an instant-read thermometer inserted into center of loaf registers 160°F.

Per serving: carbohydrates: 5 grams; Net Carbs: 3 grams; fiber: 2 grams; protein: 35 grams; fat: 23 grams; calories: 380

► Olé Turkey Tacos

Green salsa is lower in carbs than red salsa and is just as tasty. Low carb tortillas bring traditional Mexican favorites back to your table.

Prep time: 10 minutes
Cook time: 10 minutes
4 servings

2 tablespoons plus 1 teaspoon olive oil, divided
1 pound turkey cutlets
1 tablespoon chili powder
¼ cup sour cream
¼ cup chopped green onion
2 tablespoons chopped cilantro
4 low carb tortillas
½ bell pepper (any color), cut into thin strips
¼ cup sugar-free green salsa

1. Heat 1 tablespoon of oil in a large skillet. Sprinkle turkey cutlets with chili powder; cook 2 minutes per side or just until cooked through. Transfer turkey to a cutting board and cut into strips.

2. Add sour cream, green onion, and cilantro· to skillet. Cook 1 minute, stirring, until heated through. Return turkey strips and juices to skillet.

3. To crisp each tortilla, place 1 teaspoon of oil in a medium skillet and heat until very hot. Fry tortillas 1

minute per side. Fill each with ¼ of the filling. Top
with ¼ of the pepper strips and 1 tablespoon of salsa.

*Per serving: carbohydrates: 15.5 grams; Net Carbs: 5
grams; fiber: 10 grams; protein: 31 grams; fat:
20 grams; calories: 347*

➤ Chicken and Egg Salad

We've combined two favorite brunch salads in one in this recipe, and added a touch of Old Bay® seasoning for a little extra zip.

Prep time: 10 minutes
Cook time: 10 minutes
4 servings

1 tablespoon olive oil
1¼ pounds boneless skinless chicken breast, cut into
    ½-inch dice
¾ teaspoon salt, divided
5 tablespoons mayonnaise
2 tablespoons finely chopped red onion
1 tablespoon white wine vinegar
¼ teaspoon Old Bay® seasoning
2 large hard-boiled eggs
⅔ cup finely diced celery including some
    leaves

1. Heat oil in 12-inch skillet over high heat; add chicken, sprinkle with ¼ teaspoon salt and sauté, stirring as chicken browns, 5 to 7 minutes. Cool to just slightly warm.

2. Meanwhile, combine mayonnaise, onion, vinegar, remaining salt and seasoning in large bowl.

3. Finely chop eggs; stir into mayonnaise mixture with celery. Fold in chicken. Serve immediately or chill if desired.

Per serving: carbohydrates: 5 grams; Net Carbs: 4.5 grams; fiber: 0.5 grams; protein: 32 grams; fat: 23 grams; calories: 362

➤ Zucchini and Swiss Cheese Frittata

To oven-proof your skillet, wrap the handle in a double layer of aluminum foil. We used marjoram, a similar but more delicate flavor than oregano, to season the zucchini.

Prep time: 10 minutes
Cook time: 10 minutes
4 servings

2 tablespoons butter
2 medium zucchini, cut into ¼-inch rounds (2½ cups)
1 teaspoon marjoram
10 large eggs
¼ cup water
½ teaspoon salt
¾ cup coarsely shredded Swiss cheese

1. Melt butter in 12-inch nonstick ovenproof skillet over medium-high heat. Add zucchini and sauté 8 minutes; stir in marjoram. Cook just 1 to 2 minutes more until tender.

2. Meanwhile, arrange oven rack 6 inches from heat source; heat broiler. Whisk the eggs, water and salt in a bowl. Melt remaining tablespoon butter in skillet; pour eggs over squash. Reduce heat to medium-low, cover and cook until set on bottom and edges (but top will

still be loose), about 3 minutes. Sprinkle cheese evenly over top.

3. Broil frittata until just set, about 1 minute. Cut into wedges.

Per serving: carbohydrates: 4.5 grams; Net Carbs: 3 grams; fiber: 1.5 grams; protein: 23 grams; fat: 25.5 grams; calories: 343

▶ Chocolate Mudslide

Halfway between a drink and a frozen dessert, this sweet treat can be enjoyed with a spoon or slurped through a straw.

Prep time: 5 minutes
Cook time: 5 minutes
4 servings

1 cup heavy cream
½ cup water
½ cup Atkins™ Sugar Free Chocolate Syrup
2 tablespoons cocoa powder
2 teaspoons chocolate extract
1 teaspoon vanilla extract

1. In a medium saucepan, combine cream, water, syrup and cocoa. Bring to a boil over medium heat. Reduce heat to low; cook, stirring occasionally, 5 minutes. Remove from heat. Stir in chocolate and vanilla extracts.

2. Pour mixture into an 8-inch square pan. Freeze until almost solid, about 3 hours. To serve, transfer mixture to blender or food processor and blend until softened. Transfer to glasses.

Per serving: carbohydrates: 3.5 grams; Net Carbs: 2.5 grams; fiber: 0.9 grams; protein: 1.8 grams; fat: 22.4 grams; calories: 220

► Vanilla Flan

The simple flavors of vanilla, cream and eggs, gently cooked, produce a comforting and creamy dessert. Once you're past Induction, you can top these flans with berries.

Prep time: 5 minutes
Cook time: 1 hour
Chill time: 2 hours
4 servings

1 cup heavy or whipping cream
⅔ cup water
4 tablespoons granular sugar substitute
1 teaspoon vanilla extract
2 eggs
4 custard cups

1. Heat oven to 325°F. In a small saucepan, bring cream, water and sugar substitute to a simmer. Remove from heat. Stir in vanilla. Let stand 15 minutes.

2. In a medium bowl, beat eggs; gradually whisk in about one third of the cream mixture. Return egg-cream mixture to the saucepan and whisk again briefly.

3. Pour mixture through a strainer into four 6-ounce ramekins or custard cups. Place cups in a large roasting pan; carefully pour enough boiling water into pan to reach halfway up sides of cups. Cover entire pan with

foil. Bake 40 minutes, until custard is set in centers. Let cups stand in pan at room temperature 15 minutes.

4. Remove cups and cover with plastic wrap (stretch plastic over cup edges to avoid touching surface of custard). Refrigerate 2 hours, or until cold.

Per serving: carbohydrates: 2.5 grams; Net Carbs: 2.5 grams; fiber: 0 grams; protein: 4 grams; fat: 20 grams; calories: 265

PART FOUR

Beyond Induction

13 ► Phase 2—
Ongoing Weight Loss

Whether you move to the second phase of the Atkins Nutritional Approach™ (ANA) after two weeks on Induction or stay on Induction for six months, this step is key to personalizing Atkins to your needs and tastes. And while Induction takes weight off relatively quickly, you deliberately slow your weight loss in Ongoing Weight Loss, known informally as OWL.

► On OWL You Will:

- Continue to burn and dissolve fat.
- Maintain control of your appetite sufficiently to control cravings.
- Learn your threshold for carbohydrate consumption, which will allow you to continue to lose weight.
- Eat a broader range of healthy foods, selecting those that you enjoy most.

- Learn to make the most nutrient-rich choices among carbohydrate foods.
- Deliberately slow your rate of weight loss to lay the groundwork for permanent weight management.

► How Is OWL Similar to Induction?

- You will still derive the majority of your carbohydrates from vegetables low in carbs.
- You continue to burn fat for energy.
- The quality of the carbohydrate foods is as important as the quantity.
- You choose carb foods that continue to keep your blood sugar and insulin levels stable.

► How Does OWL Differ from Induction?

- You will consume more carbohydrates.
- You have more choices, so you can craft a weight-loss program that is yours alone.
- You add more portions of vegetables.
- You will slowly change the ratio of carbs to fat and protein.
- You will probably be able to gradually add nuts and seeds.
- You will probably be able to add berries.
- You will probably be able to add fresh cheeses, such as cottage and farmer cheese.

- You might be able to add other fruits, legumes or whole grains (although most people cannot in this phase).

Over the course of the next few weeks or months in this phase, you will explore a whole new way of healthy eating that will help form the parameters of your lifetime program. You'll find out how much carbohydrate consumption you can tolerate while still losing weight and continuing to control your appetite. During this phase it is a particularly good idea to keep a food diary to monitor the impact of certain foods on your appetite. Once you learn how your body reacts and how quickly you can add new foods without interfering with weight loss, you will have the tools with which to enjoy a lifetime of slimness.

▶ Finding Your Carb Threshold

When you do Atkins, your rate of weight loss is generally proportional to the amount of carbohydrate you consume. Once you know the number of grams of Net Carbs in a certain food, you know how much you can safely eat. Fortunately, counting is easy with the help of a carbohydrate gram counter. *Dr. Atkins' New Carbohydrate Gram Counter* lists grams of Net Carbs as well as total carbs for more than 1,300 common foods.

Your daily threshold of carbohydrate consumption is called your Critical Carbohydrate Level for Losing (CCLL). Stay below this number and you will experi-

ence ongoing weight loss. Exceed it and weight loss
stalls.

Here's how you'll determine your CCLL:

1. Each week, you'll incrementally increase the
   daily quantity of carbohydrate you eat beyond
   what was allowed during Induction.
2. These increments should measure roughly 5
   daily grams of Net Carbs per week, represent-
   ing one "level."

THE FIRST WEEK ON OWL

- Increase your daily Net Carb intake to 25
  grams—going up one level.
- This can be in the form of another salad, half
  an avocado, a cup of cauliflower or six to eight
  stalks of asparagus or another vegetable, or a
  controlled carb alternative food product.
- Continue to eat this way for the rest of the week.
- At the end of the week, if you have lost weight,
  you may move up another level—to 30 grams
  of Net Carbs daily—the following week.

THE SECOND WEEK ON OWL

- Increase your daily Net Carb intake to 30
  grams.
- If you like vegetables, continue to add more
  salad greens and other vegetables.

- Or add a half cup of cottage cheese, an ounce of sunflower seeds or a dozen macadamia nuts.
- Or add some berries (13 average-size strawberries contain 5 grams of carbs).
- At the end of the week, if you have lost some weight, you may move up another level—to 35 grams of Net Carbs daily—the following week.

THE THIRD WEEK ON OWL AND BEYOND

- Increase your daily Net Carb intake to 35 grams daily.
- Continue to add new foods one at a time.
- Very few people can add back all the carbohydrate food groups (particularly legumes, whole grains, fruits other than berries and starchy vegetables) during OWL.
- Continue to go up another level each week, adding another 5 daily grams of Net Carbs until you find you have lost no weight in a week.
- Drop back 5 daily grams of Net Carbs the following week.
- Weight loss should resume.
- You have found your CCLL. Above it, you lose no more, or you begin to gain. Below it, you continue to lose.
- The higher your resistance to weight loss, the lower your CCLL will be. If you are a slow loser, you may need to adjust by 5-gram increments only every two or three weeks.

► **Proceed with Caution!**

Once you decide to move to phase two, it is important
not to cut loose and undo all the good work you completed in Induction. As you learn how to liberalize that
regimen, you will be reentering the real world. That
doesn't have to be the world of junk food and uncon-
trollable cravings, but it is a world of greater choice,
and certainly one in which you will be closer to the
place where weight gain is a possibility.

What to Expect:
- You will continue to slim down, but there will
  be a gradual decrease in the rate at which you
  drop pounds and inches.
- The more slowly you lose weight, the more
  likely you are to learn healthy eating habits,
  which will help you maintain your goal weight.
  Remember that new habits take time to become
  ingrained.

Pitfalls to Avoid:
- Do not return to eating foods full of sugar,
  bleached flour and other nutrient-deficient
  carbs.
- If you add carb foods too quickly, you will stop
  your fat-burning engine. The result? Weight
  loss will cease or stall, and your cravings and
  hunger will return.

How to Get Back on Track:
- If this happens as soon as you move to OWL, return to Induction for a few days to kick-start your metabolism again and to re-establish control.
- Once you start losing again, return to OWL, this time moving more cautiously.

THE RULES OF OWL

To be successful on the second phase of Atkins, remember to follow these 15 rules:

1. Keep protein and fat as the mainstays of your diet.
2. Count your daily grams of Net Carbs.
3. Read food labels.
4. Use a carb gram counter.
5. Increase your daily Net Carb intake by no more than 5 grams each week.
6. Increase your Net Carb intake only if you continue to lose weight.
7. If you gain weight or stop losing, drop back by 5 daily grams of Net Carbs a week until weight loss resumes.
8. Add only one new food group at a time.
9. Eat a food group no more than three times per week to start, and then eat it daily.
10. Stop eating new foods immediately if they lead to weight gain or cause the return of physical symptoms lost during Induction.

11. Stop new foods if they lead to increased appetite or cravings.
12. Continue to drink eight 8-ounce glasses of water a day.
13. Continue to take a good multivitamin/mineral and an essential fatty acids supplement.
14. Continue your exercise regimen.
15. Continue doing OWL until you have 5 to 10 pounds left to lose.

14 ▶ Phase 3—
Pre-Maintenance

Many people skip this crucial phase and jump right from losing weight on Induction or OWL to trying to maintain it on Lifetime Maintenance. Almost without exception, they are headed for trouble. The Pre-Maintenance phase is *crucial* to learning the good eating habits that will allow you to maintain your goal weight once you attain it, while enhancing your health and sense of well-being.

By the time you switch to Pre-Maintenance, you're so close to your goal weight that you can almost taste it! Just 5 to 10 pounds to go, and all your problems will be solved, right? Unfortunately, it's not quite that easy.

- **Take it slowly.** Much as you may be tempted to say, "I can drop these last pounds fast now that I know how to do Atkins," you actually should do just the opposite. The fact is that the closer you get to your goal, the more slowly you should proceed. Impatient as you may be to slip easily into that new pair of jeans, you are more likely to be able to keep the weight off if you take this second to last phase of Atkins very slowly, so slowly in fact that your weight loss is almost imperceptible. It may be excruciating to move so slowly when the end is in sight. But remember: Reaching your goal weight is not your true goal. The real objective is to maintain that wonderful weight indefinitely. Once your new eating habits are ingrained, as they are more likely to be if you have more time to get used to them, the more likely they are to become habits for a lifetime.

- **Focus on the future.** You know now that you can and will reach your goal weight. The big question is whether you'll be able to maintain that weight for life. The purpose of Pre-Maintenance is to create a lifetime eating program that suits you so well that you will want to stay on it—indefinitely.

- **Half a pound a week.** The more you learn about eating as you lose those last few pounds, the better. You will now increase your carbohydrate consumption by increments of 10 grams of Net Carbs until you're losing less than a pound a week. The additional foods will provide increased nutrition and culinary enjoyment. Ideally, you should spend at least a month, and preferably two or three, in this phase.

- **Ease into Lifetime Maintenance.** By following this approach, when you reach your goal weight, you will, in effect, be on Lifetime Maintenance. During Pre-Maintenance, you will both accustom yourself to your lifetime eating plan and get a good indication of what it will be like. Think of Pre-Maintenance as a learner's permit, where you can drive only with a licensed driver by your side. You're out there doing it, but you still need some more hours behind the wheel before you're ready to be on the highway all by yourself.

- **Not the same thing.** Just because Pre-Maintenance and Lifetime Maintenance sound alike, don't make the mistake of thinking that they are the same thing. One is a training program; the other is the rest of your life. Do not skip this third phase and go right to Lifetime Maintenance. In fact, Pre-Maintenance is mandatory if you expect to achieve permanent weight loss. That way, by the time you reach your goal weight you will know exactly how you will be eating for the rest of your life—and controlling your carb intake will become automatic.

▶ The Bridge Phase

Pre-Maintenance bridges the processes of losing and maintaining weight, by helping you:

- Find your adjusted Critical Carbohydrate Level for Losing (CCLL), which should increase slightly as you deliberately slow down the loss of your last few excess pounds.
- Find your Atkins Carbohydrate Equilibrium (ACE) once you have reached your goal weight.
- Add back new foods such as legumes, fruits, and moderate amounts of whole grains and starchy vegetables into your regimen without abusing them.
- Internalize your responses to food so that what used to be a struggle with temptation becomes a deliberate and empowering choice.
- Find out how very flexible doing Atkins can be.
- Learn how to avoid making unhealthy food choices that could lead to regaining weight and beginning the yo-yo process of weight gain and loss all over again.
- Develop a style of eating that will keep you slim and vigorous for a lifetime.
- Learn which foods remain problematic for you. You will likely have to avoid them altogether or eat them rarely so that they don't interfere with your success.

THE RULES OF PRE-MAINTENANCE

To ensure success during the third phase of Atkins, follow these 15 rules:

1. Increase your daily Net Carb intake by no more than 10 grams each week so long as you continue to lose weight.
2. Be sure to continue eating adequate amounts of fat and protein even as the proportion of each diminishes slightly as part of your overall diet.
3. Continue to count your daily intake of grams of Net Carbs.
4. Continue to use a carb gram counter.
5. Continue to read food labels.
6. Add only one new food group at a time.
7. Eat a food group no more than three times per week to start, and then add it daily if possible.
8. Introduce new carb foods individually.
9. Eliminate a new food if it provokes weight gain.
10. Likewise, stop eating a new food if it prompts the return of physical symptoms lost during Induction or leads to increased appetite or cravings.
11. If you gain weight or fail to continue to lose, drop back in increments of 5 daily grams of Net Carbs a week until weight loss resumes.

12. Continue to drink eight 8-ounce glasses of water a day.
13. Continue to take a good multivitamin/mineral and an essential fatty acids supplement.
14. Continue your exercise regimen.
15. Stay on Pre-Maintenance until you have maintained your goal weight for at least one month.

15 ► Phase 4— Lifetime Maintenance

The name says it all. The fourth and final phase of Atkins allows you to maintain your goal weight for the rest of your life. The other side of the coin is that you cannot lose the weight and return to your old way of eating, and the pounds pile on again.

While you are in Pre-Maintenance, you discover your threshold for carb consumption, called your Atkins Carbohydrate Equilibrium (ACE), the number of grams of Net Carbs you can eat without gaining or losing weight. So long as you stay right at or around that number in phase four, your weight should not fluctuate beyond the perfectly natural range of 2 to 5 pounds.

Depending upon your metabolism, you will be able to eat many of the healthful foods you used to enjoy—in moderation. But sugar, beverages full of corn syrup, and other junk food made with bleached flour, sugar and trans fats remain off-limits. If you occasionally indulge in a sweet treat, get right back on track the next day, so that such behavior remains an exception to the rule rather than a return to old bad habits.

Maintaining weight loss is as much a mental challenge as a physical one. In order to continue your success for a lifetime, you need to re-create the attitude that allowed you to finally take control and lose weight.

Many of us reach for sugar and starchy foods for comfort, when proper food choices can actually lessen the impact of stress on your body. Develop strategies for dealing with temptation. Don't use food to alleviate stress or to cheer yourself up. Find ways other than food to "treat" yourself. Similarly, you'll need coping mechanisms for holidays and special occasions, as well as knowing how to get restaurants to serve you exactly what you want. For example, before you attend an event or go on a vacation where you know you will be tempted to indulge, you might decrease your carb intake so you can cut yourself a little slack later.

FALLING OFF THE WAGON

If a holiday or other event leads to a bout of unrestrained indulgence—or if you simply start eating too many carbs again—instead of waiting, act immediately! Your best opportunity to change is now—don't put it off.

- Above all, don't get depressed and give up.
- Even if you do temporarily get off track, continue to exercise and take your supplements. It's crucial that you don't surrender all control.

- Drop back by 10 daily grams of Net Carbs and see if that gets your weight loss moving again. If not, you may need to drop back further to get your fat-burning engine going. This allows you to restabilize your blood chemistry and moderate cravings so that you can be in control.
- Exercising more vigorously after going overboard will also help get you back on the straight and narrow.

▶ Be Food Smart

Remember that fresh fish, fowl, meat, and nutrient-dense carbohydrates, such as vegetables, nuts, seeds and occasional fruits and starches, are the foods nature intended you to eat, not the packaged, refined stuff. Once you're happy eating healthy foods, your nutritional future is almost assuredly going to be a healthy one. Try new foods to increase the variety of foods that you like and to avoid boredom. They will help prevent you from going back to eating foods that you have enjoyed in the past, but which simply aren't good for you.

Take care of weight regain promptly by dropping back one or more levels in daily grams of Net Carb intake until you start losing again. Once you have gotten back to your goal weight, remain at your Atkins Carbohydrate Equilibrium (ACE).

A CHANGE IN METABOLISM

As we get older, our metabolism tends to slow down a bit, making it harder to maintain the slim body many of us were blessed with in our youth. This means that the ACE you had in your thirties may not be the ACE you will be dealing with in your forties, and it is almost definitely not the ACE you'll have in the decades after that. As you age, you may eventually have to control your carb intake a little more or increase your activity level— perhaps even both—to maintain your goal weight. A change in activity level, hormone status or certain drugs also may slow your metabolism and require you to trim your carb intake.

► The Secret of Lifetime Success

Following Lifetime Maintenance can ensure not just a healthy weight but also a reduction in long-term risks for disease. This is the only body you've got. Keep it feeling and looking good. Sadly, most people who go on weight-loss diets regain all or most of their hard-lost pounds within five years. Many people even gain a few additional pounds. Don't be one of them. When you permanently change what you eat and never allow yourself to gain more than five pounds, you can truly beat the battle of the bulge.

THE RULES OF LIFETIME MAINTENANCE

Follow these 15 rules for permanent success:

1. Make your weight control and health a constant priority in your life, just as you do other things of importance in your life.
2. Continue to eat natural, unprocessed, nutrient-dense carbohydrates.
3. Continue to avoid sugar, corn syrup, honey, bleached flour and cornstarch. Read labels of any packaged food religiously and avoid any with these ingredients.
4. Regularly trying new foods and new recipes will alleviate boredom. See *www.atkins.com* for recipes suitable for all phases of Atkins.
5. Use low carb alternatives to high carb foods.
6. Learn your Atkins Carbohydrate Equilibrium (ACE) and stick to it.
7. Continue your program of vitamin and mineral supplementation, including essential oils.
8. Continue to drink at least eight 8-ounce glasses of water a day.
9. Consume caffeine and alcohol only in moderation.
10. Never let yourself gain back more than five pounds over your goal weight.
11. Don't fall back on your former bad habits.
12. Develop strategies for dealing with everyday challenges such as dining out and taking vacations.

13. Make exercise a regular part of your life.
14. Get rid of your "fat" wardrobe.
15. Weigh yourself at least once a week.

Stick to these rules and you will almost assuredly maintain your newfound weight for a lifetime!

PART FIVE

Frequently Asked Questions

► Beverages

► Can I consume alcohol on Atkins?

You should not drink alcohol during Induction, but you can drink moderate amounts during the Ongoing Weight Loss, Pre-Maintenance and Lifetime Maintenance phases of the Atkins Nutritional Approach™. Given the choice, your body will burn alcohol for energy before it burns fat. But alcohol does not act as a carbohydrate, so it will not interfere with burning fat in the same way that sugars and other carbohydrates do, although it can still interfere with weight loss if you have more than one or two drinks.

Alcohol consumption may also increase yeast-related symptoms, such as bloating, gas and cravings for sweets, and can therefore interfere with weight loss in those who are yeast sensitive. Beer, scotch and other grain-based spirits, which contain yeast, are more likely to promote yeast problems.

If it does not slow your weight loss, an occasional

glass of wine or vodka is acceptable once you are out of Induction, so long as you count the carbohydrates in your daily tally. Do not use mixers, such as juice, tonic water or non-diet soda, all of which contain sugar. Seltzer, diet tonic and non-aspartame diet soda mixers are permitted. If you have added alcohol to your regimen and suddenly stop losing weight, discontinue your alcohol intake.

▶ **Is it okay to drink light beer, which is lower in grams of carbohydrates?**

If you have yeast-related problems, such as bloating, gas, a coated tongue or cravings for sugar, you should limit beer or eliminate it from your diet. Otherwise, after Induction, you can drink light beer as long as it does not make you gain weight or stall your weight-loss efforts.

▶ **How many carbs does alcohol contain?**

It varies by type of alcoholic drink. In the case of beer, read the label. There are now a few brands of low carb beer that contain 3 grams of carbs per 12-ounce serving. For wine and spirits, refer to a carbohydrate gram counter. A 3½-ounce glass of white wine usually contains about 0.8 grams of carbs. You should not consume any alcoholic beverages during Induction.

► **Can I drink milk when doing Atkins?**

No. Milk is not permitted in the weight-loss phases because it contains too many carbohydrates, including lactose, a natural sugar. If you're craving milk, try diluting heavy cream or half-and-half with water as a substitute. Although cream is almost 100 percent fat, it does contain some lactose, so most people need to limit their intake to a maximum of 4 ounces daily to lose weight. (Be sure to count the carbs.) If you're not losing weight as quickly as you'd like, limit cream intake to no more than 2 ounces daily. Also look for alternatives, like Hood Carb Countdown™ Dairy Beverages.

► **Can I drink soymilk, almond milk or oat milk?**

All three are usually high in carbohydrates, in part because they contain added sugars. However, some manufacturers now produce soymilk with a lower carb count—check package labels to find acceptable brands. Moo Not™ Soy Milk Powder, for example, contains only 1 gram of Net Carbs per cup.

► **Can I drink diet soda while doing Atkins?**

Spring, mineral or filtered tap water and herbal teas are your best fluid options. If you must have soda, avoid caffeinated colas and look for brands, such as Diet Rite™, that are sweetened with sucralose.

▶ **How much water should I be drinking?**

On any eating regimen, the usual recommendation is a minimum of 64 ounces, or eight 8-ounce glasses, of water per day. Many people, particularly women, suffer from inadequate hydration, so it is important to be diligent about drinking water throughout the day. Drinking sufficient water also will help flush toxins from your body and combat such problems as constipation and bad breath. Note that coffee, tea and diet sodas do not apply to the daily minimum. Adequate hydration also assists with weight loss.

▶ **Why is caffeine unacceptable on the Atkins Nutritional Approach™?**

Excess caffeine can drop blood sugar levels and leave you craving sweets. If you're addicted to caffeine, you must minimize caffeine consumption. The best way to do this is to segue from the high-octane stuff to decaf by gradually adding decaf to your full-force brew until you are drinking straight decaf, which you can enjoy with cream. Water-processed decaf is preferable because it does not use chemicals, as other decaffeinating processes do. If you are not addicted to caffeine, you can probably still have one cup of regular coffee a day without experiencing cravings. Remember that most cola drinks also contain caffeine.

▶ **Can I drink flavored coffees?**

Some flavored coffees contain hidden carbohydrates in the form of sugar or corn syrup. Hazelnut, almond, or other nut- or grain-extracted (decaf) flavors are fine, but do check labels for the carb count. You can also add Atkins™ Sugar Free Chocolate, Hazelnut or Vanilla Syrup to decaf coffee if you're looking for more flavor without added sugar. Some of these syrups are also good in decaffeinated tea.

▶ **Can I drink tomato and other vegetable juices on Induction?**

No. When the fiber is removed and there is a more concentrated source of the vegetable, as in juice, it may have a more profound impact on blood sugar and therefore should be avoided on Induction. Most vegetable juices are acceptable in later phases.

▶ Children and Teenagers

▶ **Can children or teenagers do Atkins?**

The number of children and teens who are overweight or obese has reached epidemic proportions. The Atkins Nutritional Approach™ can be followed by children and teens if it is recommended by a physician who also monitors the program to ensure that the proper foods and supplements are consumed and that

weight loss does not occur too rapidly, which could
stunt growth. But remember, young children tend to
eat the way their parents do. That's why it's important
the whole family eat healthy, balanced meals. We suggest that you cut out sugar, processed food, junk food
and other refined carbohydrates. The earlier parents in-
still good nutritional habits, the healthier their children
will be—now and in the future. You can also set a good
example by being physically fit.

► Fiber

► How can I get adequate fiber while doing Atkins?

Fiber is found in plant-based foods, such as fruit,
vegetables, whole grains, nuts and seeds. A tablespoon
or two of wheat bran, psyllium husks or ground
flaxseed will meet your fiber requirements during Induction when your carbohydrate intake is limited to
three cups of vegetables daily (it can also help relieve
constipation, which may occur during this period). You
don't have to count the carbs in fiber because they have
a negligible impact on blood sugar levels. Keep in
mind: Fiber supplements must be taken with plenty of
water. You can also try Atkins Fiber Drops™, an
orange-flavored hard candy and fiber supplement all in
one with more than 2 grams of fiber per piece.

▶ **How do you deal with fiber when calculating Net Carbs?**

Consuming fiber will not interfere with weight loss because it has a negligible impact on blood sugar levels. So to get the Net Carb count, simply subtract the number of grams of fiber from the grams of total carbohydrates.

▶ **Doesn't the limited number of servings of vegetables and omission of fruit on Atkins fail to provide enough dietary fiber?**

The Induction phase of Atkins does not quite meet the United States Department of Agriculture requirements for intake of fiber, which is 25 to 35 grams daily. This can easily be met by supplementing your diet with a tablespoon or more of wheat bran, psyllium husks or flax meal. Once you add more vegetables, berries, seeds and nuts back into your diet, you will be consuming plenty of fiber.

▶ **Can I use Metamucil® on Atkins?**

Yes, but check the label to be sure to purchase the sugar-free variety.

► Fitness and Exercise

► When it comes to athletic endurance, will following the Atkins Nutritional Approach™ affect my performance?

It is a misconception that carb-loading is the best way to prepare yourself for endurance exercise. Although an overabundance of carbs might give you an initial burst of energy, that surge can then lead to a sharp drop in your blood sugar—resulting in fatigue—later in your workout. This isn't to say that you should eliminate all carbs from your diet, but endurance athletes will do better by consuming moderate amounts of nutrient-dense, unrefined carbohydrates, found in foods such as kale, spinach and broccoli, nuts and seeds and low glycemic fruits to ensure a stable blood sugar throughout a workout. For more information on training and nutrition, visit *www.atkins.com*.

► Do I need to exercise to lose weight on Atkins?

You may be able to lose weight without exercising, but it is not recommended. Exercise not only speeds weight loss, helps maintain a healthy weight and enhances muscle tone, it also offers a host of other health benefits, like a reduced risk of heart disease, stroke, high blood pressure, colon cancer and Type 2 diabetes. Weight-bearing exercise is also essential to maintain bone mass in men and women, especially as we age.

➤ How long does it take to see results from exercise?

Be patient. Two weeks is not enough time for exercise to change your body. Some people, especially those who are flabby, may even gain a little weight. That's because muscle mass increases as you get stronger, and muscle is denser than fat. From our thirties on, we begin to lose muscle mass. That's one reason your metabolic rate slows down as you age. The more muscle you have, the more oxygen you take in; oxygen burns fat, so in turn, you burn more fat. If you follow an exercise program five days a week, you should see results within a month.

➤ What kind of exercise do I need, and what's the best way to get started?

You need a combination of aerobic exercise, for its cardiovascular benefits, and weight-bearing exercise, to protect your bones and strengthen your muscles as you age. For this reason, it is particularly important that women establish a regular exercise program.

Check with your doctor before embarking on a new exercise routine. Then, start with any aerobic exercise at any level you can sustain. (If you are overweight, don't start off running; it places too much stress on your body.) If you're out of shape and very heavy, you may start with only 10 minutes of exercise a day. Such exercise might consist of chair exercises or water aerobics. Just make sure to engage in that 10-minute regimen each day. The body can usually handle a 10 percent increase in workload per week.

It's also a good idea to vary your workouts so you don't get bored. For example, you might ride a bicycle twice a week and walk the other days. Another important motivation for exercising is the knowledge that the more muscle you have, the more fat you will burn. That's because muscles carry oxygen and oxygen burns fat.

The most recent U.S. Surgeon General's Report on Physical Activity and Health recommends at least 60 minutes each day of moderately intense physical activity to prevent weight gain and reap the full health benefits of activity. Eventually, you should be exercising for one hour a day.

▶ **What kind of exercise is safe for extremely overweight people?**

People who are very heavy, regardless of age, should never start an exercise program without consulting their physician. If you get the okay, do not start with an exercise program that stresses muscles and joints, such as running, tennis or skiing. Instead, walking, riding a stationary bike and swimming are all good choices. You can also do chair exercises, perhaps with bands that provide resistance. If you choose to swim, a great way to exercise is to use buoyancy vests or belts that make it easy to do water aerobics.

Always remember to drink plenty of water when exercising. If you're not thirsty and not sweating noticeably, you still need to increase your intake of fluids, even when exercising outdoors in cold weather. Aside from its other detrimental effects on the body, dehydration causes more lactic acid buildup and more soreness in the muscles.

The important thing is to get moving, no matter how little at the beginning. As exercise becomes part of your routine, you will feel better and find it increasingly enjoyable and empowering.

► Food and Eating Behavior

► **My weight varies by a few pounds every day. Why is this?**

It's natural for your weight to vary from day to day, mostly due to your fluid intake, which is why we discourage weighing yourself every day. (Your weight may also vary from morning to evening, so be sure to weigh yourself at the same time of day each time.) From week to week, you should be seeing a difference in the way your clothes fit. For added incentive we encourage taking body measurements at the start of the program and every two weeks thereafter.

► **As long as I stay at 20 grams of Net Carbs a day during Induction, why can't I have some carbohydrates in the form of whole-grain bread or a chocolate bar?**

There are two reasons this approach won't work. For one, all carbohydrates are not created equal. The Atkins Nutritional Approach™ is designed to prevent blood sugar levels from spiking and causing the over-production of insulin—a hormone that helps convert carbohydrates to body fat. The first carbohydrates you need to add back to your diet when you move beyond Induction are vegetables, then seeds and nuts, then berries, and then—if you are still losing—legumes and grains. Even bread made from 100 percent whole-wheat flour contains enough refined carbs to produce this insulin-raising, fat-storing effect in many people. Later, if your weight loss is progressing well and you have increased your daily carb intake, you may eat an occasional slice of whole-grain bread.

Second, Atkins is not just about rapid weight loss—it's about learning to eat only nutrient-dense carbohydrates for the rest of your life. These are foods that are packed with the most antioxidant vitamins and health-ful phytochemicals relative to the amount of carbohydrates—so you're getting the most bang for your carbohydrate buck. Once you are close to your goal weight and are close to establishing your personal Atkins Carbohydrate Equilibrium (ACE), if you are like most people, you will be able to enjoy a slice of whole-grain bread, half a banana or even the occasional baked potato. You can, however, enjoy a slice of Atkins Bakery™ Ready-to-Eat Sliced Bread even during Induction.

▶ Why are there discrepancies in carb counts from label to label and from book to book?

You will see inconsistencies because carbohydrates cannot be measured as accurately as fats and protein can be. On food labels, the number of carb grams indicated is basically what is left over after the fats and protein (as well as water and ash) are analytically assayed for weight. So when you back into the number of carbohydrate grams, the variance allowed in assays of other components can be compounded in the carbohydrate count. Moreover, the Food and Drug Administration allows a 20 percent margin of error on reporting Class II nutrients (including carbohydrates) on a product label.

When it comes to carb counts listed in books, there are several additional factors that come into play. The quality of the data entered is obviously a factor, as is the process by which the calculations are made. In the case of whole foods, such as broccoli, the following variations could affect the total count: Is the broccoli cooked or raw? Do the florets include their stems or not? Is the quantity loosely packed or crammed into a cup? Moreover, some books list servings without specifying exactly what that constitutes. Additionally, there is more than one form of computer software used for analysis and each may provide somewhat different results. These systems also still have some "bugs" in them, causing variations in the analysis. In the case of packaged foods, the inconsistencies mentioned above also come into play.

Finally, most labels do not distinguish Net Carbs, which are the only grams of carbs you need to count when you do Atkins. In the most basic terms, Net Carbs are total grams of carbohydrate minus grams of fiber, which have negligible impact on blood sugar.

▶ **What is the difference between soy powder, soy protein isolate, soy flour, protein powder and whey protein isolate, and which are low in carbs?**

Soy (also called soya) powder and soy flour are both made from soybeans. Both contain protein and some carbohydrate and are appropriate for doing Atkins. Soy powder is ground finer than soy flour and therefore works better in shakes; soy flour, used for baking, is denser than soy powder and therefore has more carbs. For best results, especially in the Induction phase, use Atkins Quick Quisine™ Bake Mix, which has a very low carb count, instead of soy flour, when baking.

Soy protein isolate, as the name implies, separates the protein from the carbohydrate content of the soybean, making it lower in carbs than either soy flour or soy powder.

Protein powder is a source of pure protein, usually an egg protein or vegetable-based protein powder. Keep in mind that many protein powders contain certain carb-laden fillers and hidden sugars. Make sure you read the label to check carbohydrate and sugar content.

Whey protein isolate (WPI) is considered the highest-quality protein available in terms of the body's ability to utilize it. It is extremely low in carbohydrates, high in protein and contains virtually no fat. It has also been shown to possess immune-boosting capabilities by increasing the body's cellular levels of glutathione, an important antioxidant. Atkins Advantage™ Shake Mixes and Ready-to-Drink Shakes include WPI as an ingredient.

► **What are some healthful snack ideas for feeding my children instead of the usual junk foods?**

Try serving up blueberries with whipped cream, or a mix of nuts, seeds and raisins. Other ideas include whole-grain bread or crackers with cheese or peanut butter, celery sticks with peanut or another nut butter, popcorn made in an air popper and drizzled with melted butter, deviled eggs, rolled-up slices of turkey, or ham with cheese.

Instead of soda or fruit juice, offer kids flavored seltzers or iced herbal teas. If they're hooked on fruit juice, offer the whole fruit instead—which causes a less dramatic rise in blood sugar. In the winter, you can make hot chocolate using Splenda® instead of sugar. Also, keep a supply of Atkins Advantage™ Bars and Atkins Morning Start™ Breakfast Bars handy for snacking, and make treats from Atkins Advantage™ Shake Mix or Atkins Endulge™ Ice Cream Cups. Check out *www.atkins.com* for recipe ideas, too.

► **Since starting Atkins, I have bad breath. What can I do about it?**

When your body primarily burns fat as fuel rather than glucose, it generates ketones, the by-products of fat breakdown that are released in your breath and your urine. While this can be annoying, the good news is that "ketone breath" is chemical proof that you're burning stored body fat. The more ketones you release, the more fat you've burned.

Drinking plenty of water helps dilute the concentration of ketones. Parsley is a natural breath freshener as is oil of peppermint drops, available at health food stores. (Read the label to ensure that they contain no sugar.) Chewing fresh parsley or taking capsules such as BreathAsure®, which can be found in any health food or drugstore, will help. As long as you drink enough water, the bad breath caused by ketosis usually lasts only a few weeks.

▶ **Where can I find a comprehensive carbohydrate gram counter?**

Dr. Atkins' New Carbohydrate Gram Counter is a handy pocket-size booklet you can take to restaurants or the grocery store. You can also refer to the carb counter in Food & Recipes, at *www.atkins.com*.

▶ **What is the difference between a carbohydrate gram counter and a glycemic index?**

A carbohydrate gram counter typically lists the total carbohydrate value of a food item. On Atkins, however, the only carbs that matter are Net Carbs, which are provided in *Dr. Atkins' New Carbohydrate Gram Counter*. The glycemic index is a measure of how quickly a given carbohydrate raises your blood sugar level. You can use the glycemic index to choose carbohydrate foods that will have a relatively low impact on your blood sugar. But remember, when doing Atkins, your total carbohydrate intake is of utmost importance.

► **What are some ideas for brown-bag lunches that I can eat during Induction?**

Hard-boiled eggs, chicken wings or drumsticks, string cheese or other prepackaged cheese (but no artificial cheeses); and rolled-up slices of turkey, chicken, roast beef, lox (filled with cream cheese) or Swiss cheese are all ideal portable lunch foods. You can also prepare tasty sandwiches using Atkins Bakery™ Ready-to-Eat Sliced Bread and roast beef or sliced turkey, or tuna, salmon, chicken or egg salads made with mayonnaise and celery. (During Induction, make it an open-face sandwich.) Any green salad can be garnished with protein, either from a salad bar or brought from home. Condiments such as olives and avocado make salads more appealing. Invest in an insulated container and add an ice pack, or stow in the office fridge.

► **Why am I craving sweets, bread and crackers?**

If you recently started doing Atkins, your blood sugar levels probably haven't yet stabilized. After adhering strictly to Induction for five days, cravings should be under control. Occasionally, women will experience cravings just before a menstrual period. The longer you continue doing Atkins, the fewer cravings you should experience.

Skipping meals or going too long between meals also may cause cravings—one reason why eating regularly is important. Another possibility is that you may have a food allergy. People often crave the very food they should stay away from—milk products, peanuts, wheat, yeast and corn are common culprits. You will not be eating peanuts, wheat or corn on Induction. Eliminate any other suspect foods one at a time to see if the cravings abate.

Stress is another possible trigger for cravings. Blood sugar can become unstable when you're under stress, which in turn leads to cravings. Excessive caffeine can also cause a hypoglycemic response, or an unstable blood sugar level, in some individuals, which can lead to cravings for sweets. The supplement L-glutamine may help curb cravings, as does Atkins Dieters' Advantage™, which contains nutrients and food extracts that help control appetite, including chromium to help stabilize blood sugar.

Consuming fat can help you feel more satisfied, mitigating cravings. If you're doing everything else right and still craving carbs, eat one of the following: half of an Atkins Advantage™ Bar, a few olives, some cheese, avocado or some cream cheese spread on a celery stick. Most important, don't give in to cravings. Doing so will only result in more cravings and more cheating—and inevitable weight gain.

➤ **I'm having withdrawal symptoms from not eating sugar. What can I do?**

During Induction, a small percentage of people experience withdrawal symptoms, which may include headaches, nausea, dizziness, fatigue, muscle cramps or irritability. If you can ride out the symptoms, they should disappear within four or five days. Otherwise, try increasing your intake of vegetables for several days. As soon as the symptoms have abated, go back to consuming no more than 20 grams of Net Carbs a day. Be sure you are drinking enough water and taking a vitamin/mineral supplement that contains magnesium, calcium and potassium.

➤ **You can eat a lot of eggs on Atkins. Isn't all that cholesterol unhealthy?**

If we had to name a perfect food, the egg would be it. While many foods supply a handful of vitamins and minerals, eggs are nature's perfect food. The egg is one of the few foods that can provide all eight essential amino acids, the building blocks of protein (as well as choline). Since our bodies don't manufacture these eight substances, we have to get them through foods or supplements. The yolk of an egg is protein, so eating egg-white omelets, for example, means missing out on the most nutrient-dense part of the egg.

People who have avoided eggs for years, fearing their cholesterol count, can still have high blood cholesterol. When you are following a controlled carb lifestyle and are beneath your threshold of carbohydrate tolerance, you are burning fat for energy. Moreover, the cholesterol found in an egg will have no impact on your total blood cholesterol on a controlled carbohydrate nutritional approach.

► **Once I've reached my goal weight, what kinds of foods are allowed on Lifetime Maintenance?**

To a large extent, your personal carbohydrate threshold will regulate your maintenance regimen, which is a result of your metabolism and your activity level. Younger people and men tend to have higher metabolisms than older people and women. If you have a high carbohydrate threshold and do vigorous exercise on a regular basis, you may be able to regularly eat starchy vegetables, beans and other legumes, whole grains and fruit in moderation. On the other hand, if you have a low carb threshold and are not very active, you may have to stay away from many of these foods or have them only as an occasional treat. In either case, your nutrition program will continue to stress whole foods and curb sugar, bleached flour, hydrogenated fats and any processed foods.

► **Why does doing Atkins give you a metabolic advantage over low fat weight-loss programs?**

The simple answer is that it takes more energy to burn fat and protein for energy than it does to burn carbohydrate. Conventional thinking is that the number of calories you consume (and expend) determines the use or storage of that energy. Eat fewer calories and use up more of them, and you will lose weight. However, low fat, low calorie diets are not satiating and therefore hard to stay on, and their high carbohydrate content often leads to food cravings and binge eating. In contrast, by controlling the intake of carbohydrates and thus burning body fat for energy, individuals on Atkins can eat high fat, satisfying foods that contain more calories, and still lose weight. That edge is called the *metabolic advantage*.

▶ **Why must I avoid margarine?**

Natural fats are encouraged on the Atkins Nutritional Approach™, but there is an unnatural category of fats that contain compounds that do not melt at body temperature and therefore can contribute to plaque formation in the blood vessels, increasing the risk of stroke and heart disease. These processed fats, called trans fats, are found in hydrogenated oil, which includes most margarines as well as shortening, some brands of peanut butter and many processed baked goods and snack foods. We recommend butter over margarine; however, some margarines are not hydrogenated and are an acceptable alternative. The label will state "no trans fats." Other healthy fat selections include olives and olive oil, avocado, nuts and nut oils, flaxseed and flax oil, sunflower seeds and their oil, and oily fish such as salmon, sardines and mackerel. Safflower and corn oil are acceptable, but should not be a dominant source of fats. It is important to consume a balance of all types of fat, including monounsaturated, polyunsaturated and saturated fats.

▶ What are nitrates and why are they bad for you?

Nitrates and nitrites are added to meats (such as bacon and cured ham) and smoked fish to produce an appealing color and inhibit growth of germs and poisons. While these chemical compounds are not themselves carcinogens, they can yield by-products such as nitrosamines, which have been implicated in higher rates of cancer—particularly colon and gastric cancer—in animals. For this reason, it is prudent to limit your intake of foods containing nitrates or nitrites. Look for nitrate-free products in natural foods stores and some supermarkets.

▶ Will I ever be able to eat pasta again?

If you have a relatively high threshold for carbohydrate intake and are someone who is relatively active, you may be able to reincorporate moderate portions of pasta by the time you are in Pre-Maintenance or Lifetime Maintenance. If you occasionally want pasta or another carb-filled food at that point, plan for it. Cut back on your carbs for a day, then have the pasta meal that night, then cut back again the next day. If you want to eat pasta on a regular basis, have a small portion (a half cup) and enjoy it with enough fat and protein so that the sugars are released at a slower, steadier pace.

If possible, have whole-wheat or soy-based pasta instead of conventional pasta made from bleached flour. Atkins Quick Quisine™ Pasta Cuts, made from soy, with only 3 grams of Net Carbs per serving, are suitable foods once you are in Ongoing Weight Loss. Also try Atkins Quick Quisine™ Pasta Sides in three varieties: Elbows & Cheese, Fettuccine Alfredo and Pesto Cream.

▶ **Doesn't all the protein you eat on Atkins cause kidney and liver problems?**

There are no studies indicating that Atkins causes kidney or liver problems in healthy individuals. Research trials that looked at liver and kidney and heart function with participants on controlled carbohydrate diets similar to Atkins showed no negative effects. Individuals who are suffering from far-advanced kidney disease are extremely restricted in everything they consume, including water, so Atkins would not be appropriate for them.

▶ **I really miss eating fruit. Which ones are relatively low in carbs?**

You should avoid fruit completely during Induction, because most people find it interferes with fat burning. When you move to Ongoing Weight Loss, you can introduce berries, which are relatively low in carbohydrates, as long as they don't slow or stop your weight loss. A three-quarter-cup serving of fresh strawberries or raspberries or a third of a cup of fresh blueberries contains approximately 5 grams of Net Carbs.

When you reach Pre-Maintenance, most people can also enjoy low-glycemic fruits such as plums, nectarines, apples, cherries and kiwi in moderate amounts. Again, continue to count carbs and refer to your carb gram counter. You can also eat up to one cup of berries each day. Have high-sugar citrus fruits only occasionally—grapefruit is lowest—and bananas only once in a while. Avoid fruit juices, which provide huge doses of sugar (a splash to flavor seltzer is okay). Choose whole, fiber-rich fruit instead.

As a general rule, limit your fruit servings to one or two a day. After you have tested your tolerance to fruit sugar and are still able to gradually lose or maintain your weight, depending upon your phase of the program, you can try the higher glycemic fruits such as pears, mangos, melons, pineapple and so forth. Eating fruit with nuts, cheese, or whipped cream will slow down the release of the sugars into the bloodstream.

► **I thought I wasn't supposed to be hungry when I do Atkins, but I am. What gives?**

If you're hungry, eat! If you're starving, you should have eaten 30 minutes ago. Just as overeating can cause your body to resist weight loss, so can eating too little, which slows down your metabolism. Eat adequate amounts of food and eat regularly. Also, be sure to eat enough fat (the natural kinds, like olive oil, fatty fish and avocado); foods containing fat and protein are the most satiating. Not eating enough fat will also interfere with your body's ability to burn its own fat for energy.

► **Can I do a low fat version of Atkins?**

Fat is the mechanism that makes controlled carbohydrate weight loss work. The Atkins Nutritional Approach™ teaches you how to use fat to your advantage. When you are doing Atkins, fat is your friend not only because it is satiating but because it slows the release of glucose into the blood. By moderating blood sugar swings, fat reduces carbohydrate cravings. Dietary fat, in combination with controlled carbohydrate consumption, accelerates the burning of stored body fat. When your body uses fat, rather than glucose for fuel, the metabolic process is called *lipolysis*.

However, you do want to focus on "good" fats. Natural, healthy fat is found in olives and olive oil, seeds, nuts, seed and nut oils and butters, avocado, and oily fish such as salmon, sardines and mackerel. Saturated fat, found in meats, butter and coconut oil, poses no health risk when balanced with other choices of fat such as polyunsaturated and monounsaturated fats. You will burn both dietary and body fat for energy when carbohydrate consumption is controlled and you stay at or beneath your carbohydrate threshold. The kinds of fat you should avoid are chemically altered, processed hydrogenated oils, also known as trans fats, which can be found in shortening and most commercially packaged processed foods. Foods such as cookies, crackers, pretzels, potato chips, non-dairy creamers, corn chips, cereals and breads often contain trans fats. Take time to read the ingredients and avoid hydrogenated or partially hydrogenated oils. Look for cold-pressed or expeller-pressed oils, and store them in a dark, cool place to keep them from going rancid or oxidizing. High heat changes the molecular structure of the cell and will transform even a good fat into a bad fat, so be sure not to burn oil or allow it to smoke while cooking.

People who try to do their own low fat version of Atkins will not only find themselves hungry, they also will not achieve the weight-loss results of those who consume healthy fats.

▶ **Are nuts and seeds okay on Induction even though they have carbohydrates?**

Different nuts and seeds have different percentages of fat, protein and carbohydrate. We don't recommend eating them during the first two weeks of Induction. But after that, if you are continuing to lose weight steadily, you can try introducing some.

It is worth mentioning that nuts are notoriously hard to eat in moderation. One leads to another until you may have eaten several ounces. Buy the one- or two-ounce packets for built-in portion control, so you won't be tempted to overindulge.

► **I heard that people on Atkins get used to eating fatty foods like bacon and eggs, so when they go off the program, they gain even more weight. Is this true?**

No. For starters, Atkins is an eating plan designed to be followed for a lifetime. Most people become overweight because they eat sugary and other processed, refined foods and their bodies aren't able to use up those empty calories. Eating high fat foods such as eggs, cheese and a couple of pieces of bacon is fine only in the absence of excessive carbs in general and refined carbs in particular. During Induction, when carbohydrates are most severely controlled, you can indeed eat plenty of fat, all the while losing weight and improving your blood cholesterol and triglyceride markers. However, once your weight loss slows and you are no longer primarily burning fat for energy, you will naturally start to replace some of the fat in your diet with nutrient-dense carbohydrates.

In all phases of Atkins, it is a good idea to get some of your fat from fatty fish such as salmon, tuna and sardines, nuts and seeds and olive oil, which has well-documented health benefits. If you do eat bacon, look for products that are not cured with nitrates.

Second, if a person does Atkins, loses weight and then returns to his old way of high carbohydrate eating, whether or not he incorporates bacon and eggs, he will likely regain the weight. And eating a high fat, high carbohydrate diet, which is the typical American diet, is a recipe for health disaster. The point is that Atkins is a lifetime eating plan. The gradual process by which you learn new healthy eating habits actually reinforces these behaviors.

► **What should I know about studies stating that a high fat intake is detrimental to your health?**

All the studies stating that a high fat intake is detrimental to your health have been done in mixed diet settings where there was enough carbohydrate in the diet for the body to burn glucose (instead of primarily fat) for energy. When fat is the primary fuel source, you metabolize fat instead of storing it, and it poses no health risk. There are no studies that have linked low carbohydrate, high fat eating programs to any health risk.

► **Is it true that Atkins works simply because it's a low calorie diet?**

No. While some people who do Atkins may eat fewer calories than before, it is not because the program is restrictive or unduly limits food intake. They may be eating fewer calories because they are generally less hungry and less obsessed with food. On the other hand, studies show that someone doing Atkins can eat more calories than does a low fat dieter—and lose more weight. For example, a 2001 study of overweight and obese teens at Schneider Children's Hospital in New Hyde Park, New York, found that those on a high protein, high fat diet of 1,800 calories a day lost

10.5 more pounds on average than did those in a group eating a typical low fat, 1,100-calorie diet. And in the high protein group, total cholesterol and triglyceride levels dropped, while HDL ("good") cholesterol increased.

▶ **Is it true that doing Atkins makes you crave sweets?**

No. If you are addicted to sugar, doing Atkins merely makes you aware of that addiction. And the surefire way to cure any addiction is abstinence. Atkins eliminates sugar from the diet, breaking that addiction. Meanwhile, fat and protein lend a feeling of satiety, which makes you feel fuller and satisfied for longer periods. The by-products of fat burning are ketones, which have a natural appetite-suppressing effect. Cravings for sweets usually disappear after the third or fourth day on Induction, so people find they have more control over what they eat. For additional support, the supplements chromium and L-glutamine can help you overcome your addiction to sugar.

▶ **Why does Atkins allow fried foods? Aren't they unhealthy?**

Fried foods can make doing Atkins more enjoyable and they do not adversely affect fat burning. However, given a choice, broiling, roasting or sautéing meat is preferable; these cooking methods eliminate the "bad fats" that can be created by the ultra-high heat required for frying. You should never coat fried foods with flour or bread crumbs; instead, use ground nuts or seeds.

► Can a vegetarian follow the Atkins Nutritional Approach™?

While scientific research supports the advantages of consuming a diet that incorporates healthy quantities of poultry, fish, pork and beef, many individuals are committed to vegetarianism for a wide range of reasons, from philosophical to culinary motivations. Atkins is a viable option for vegetarians—especially those who consume excess starch (refined grains, pasta, potatoes, chips and other snack foods). By following a controlled carb vegetarian approach, individuals benefit from a more satisfying, nutrient-rich way of eating. Proteins, such as tofu, tempeh, seitan, eggs and cheese, nuts and seeds can be substituted for meat, poultry and fish. In addition to low-glycemic vegetables and fruits, lentils and other legumes, nuts and seeds are encouraged, depending on one's carbohydrate tolerance or Atkins Carbohydrate Equilibrium (ACE). During Induction, vegetarians should pay special attention to their fat intake, being sure to use generous amounts of oil and other fats and enjoying appropriate foods, like avocados and olives, to ensure that they are consuming enough calories. Vegetarians should also take advantage of Atkins Nutritionals' array of low carb products such as bread and pasta made from soy.

► **Why does the Atkins Nutritional Approach™ limit the amount of cheese I can eat?**

Although cheese is a source of protein and fat, unlike meat it contains carbohydrates. When you do Atkins, you can enjoy up to four ounces of cheese a day. As a rule of thumb, one ounce of aged cheese—about a 1-inch cube or ¼ cup shredded—provides 1 gram of carbohydrate and no fiber. (Aged cheeses include blue, Brie, cheddar, Edam, Gouda, Gruyère, Havarti, Jarlsberg, Parmesan, provolone, Romano and Swiss.) Fresh cheeses, like cottage cheese, farmer cheese, feta and ricotta, typically provide more grams of carbohydrate per serving. (**Note:** There is no fiber in cheese, so Net Carbs = total carbs.)

► **Can drinking tea help me lose weight?**

There is some evidence to suggest that tea may increase your metabolic rate and help marginally speed up your weight loss. A 1999 study of 10 healthy young men showed that when they took capsules containing green tea extract, their energy expenditure increased more than when they took capsules containing caffeine or just sugar. In other words, the green tea extract made their metabolisms run faster and they burned more fat.

Even if green tea has only a small effect on your metabolism, drinking it can help your weight-loss efforts in other ways. A cup of hot decaffeinated tea, along with a small protein snack, is a great way to allay between-meal hunger pangs. In addition, a cup of tea about half an hour before mealtime can help suppress your appetite and make you less likely to overeat. And instead of dessert, try having a cup of lightly sweetened tea. To keep carbs in your tea to a minimum, use a non-caloric sweetener such as Splenda® and skip the milk.

► Health and Medical Issues

► How will doing Atkins help to lower my cholesterol?

There are two sources of energy to fuel our bodies: glucose and fat. When you sufficiently restrict carbohydrates you will allow your body to predominantly burn fat for energy. When you burn dietary fat for energy, it is metabolized rather than stored and therefore poses no serious health risks. Your stored body fat also is burned. That's why not long after you start doing Atkins, a blood test will reveal a lower level of triglycerides, which will bring down your total cholesterol and raise your HDL ("good") cholesterol.

► Since beginning Atkins, I am often constipated. How can I avoid this?

Some degree of constipation is common during the first week of Induction. This is due to the change in diet, especially the reduction of fruit and vegetable fiber. Be sure that you are taking in at least three cups of salad vegetables, not using your carb allotment on other foods and drinking the minimum of eight glasses of water daily. After the first couple of weeks, your body should adjust and constipation shouldn't be a problem. And when you begin to add more carbohydrates, your first choices should be more vegetables, followed by seeds and nuts and berries. If constipation continues, there are several remedies. First, make sure you are getting those eight 8-ounce glasses of water each day. Inadequate hydration is the main reason for constipation. Most people, especially women, don't drink enough water and are slightly dehydrated much of the time. Second, consume some supplementary fiber in the form of wheat bran sprinkled on a salad, psyllium husks mixed with water or iced decaf herbal tea, or ground flaxseed blended into a protein drink. The amount needed to stay regular varies from person to person. Start with a tablespoonful. It may take a few days to find the amount that works for you. Do be careful not to use too much fiber; in excess, it can actually act as a binder. Finally, increasing physical activity often helps.

▶ **I am a diabetic. Can I follow the Atkins Nutritional Approach™?**

The ANA can actually decrease the risk for developing insulin resistance or diabetes. Controlling carbohydrate intake has also been shown to regulate blood sugar levels and insulin production, therefore diminishing the need for medications. Of course, with any medical condition such as this, close medical supervision is essential, especially if you are already taking medications. Your physician will need to adjust your dosage as you limit carb intake. Losing weight and controlling carbohydrate intake also will reverse or moderate insulin resistance. Many people are able to get off or avoid medications completely (with the exception of Type 1 diabetics); others will need to maintain a minimum dosage.

► **I've had several episodes of diarrhea since starting Atkins. How can I avoid it?**

Diarrhea is uncommon in people doing Atkins. In fact, individuals on Induction are more likely to initially experience constipation. However, some people can't tolerate dairy products—and consumption of cheese and cream may cause diarrhea. Eliminating all milk products may help. Unsweetened psyllium husks, which are a bulking agent and act as a sponge, soaking up water and helping form a normal stool, can be added to the diet. Eating more fat than you are used to also can provoke this response. Individuals who have been on an extremely low fat diet prior to starting Atkins may find it takes their body a while to adjust.

If dietary fat is not the cause, diarrhea could result from taking the recommended supplements. Try stopping them for a week, and then if the diarrhea disappears, reintroduce them one at a time. As long as you have diarrhea, it is especially important to drink a minimum of eight 8-ounce glasses of water a day so as to avoid dehydration.

> ➤ I have been experiencing dizziness since beginning Atkins. Why, and what should I do?

If you are just beginning Atkins, it is possible that you are experiencing carbohydrate withdrawal, which should last no longer than four to five days at most. Increasing your salad and other vegetable intake should ease symptoms. After several days, resume the Induction level of Net Carbs. Be sure that you are eating regularly and not skipping meals or ignoring feelings of hunger. In addition, stay well hydrated. If you have lost weight too quickly, it is possible that you have some mineral loss that needs to be replaced. Be sure you are taking a multivitamin and mineral supplement. If symptoms continue, consult your health care practitioner.

> ➤ I've heard that doing Atkins will give me more energy, but since I've started the program I feel weak and lethargic. Why, and what can I do?

If you are just beginning Atkins, you may be suffering carbohydrate withdrawal as you start the Induction phase. Headaches, irritability, nausea, dizziness and fatigue are the most common symptoms. If you have a tendency to get migraines, carbohydrate withdrawal may trigger them. If you're going to experience withdrawal, it generally starts within 12 hours of changing your diet. Fortunately, it generally doesn't last more than four or five days, although occasionally it can last up to a week.

If you're not taking a multivitamin/mineral and essential fatty acids, sometimes taking vitamin/mineral supplements is all that you need to address the fatigue.

It's important to understand that your body has been running on a glucose (sugar) metabolism all your life. Glucose is the body's preferred source of fuel because it burns fast. Doing Atkins switches you from a glucose metabolism to a primarily fat metabolism. Withdrawal occurs during the adaptation period in which that switch takes place. Until you adapt to this new fuel source, you may feel tired, have headaches or experience other symptoms.

When your body becomes accustomed to burning fat for fuel, these symptoms should go away. In the meantime, you may alleviate them by increasing your carb intake slightly. Do this by eating more vegetables such as salad greens, spinach, broccoli and string beans. Once your body adjusts and symptoms have abated, reduce your carb intake to 20 grams a day again.

One way to keep your energy up is to eat snacks rich in protein and fat throughout the day. At home, try a slice of turkey or cream cheese on celery. On the go, pack some cheese cubes or an Atkins Advantage™ Bar or Atkins Morning Start™ Breakfast Bar. After the first two weeks of Induction, nuts and seeds make excellent snacks as well.

Some people try the Atkins program for three or four days and then give up, which never gives their bodies the chance to make that metabolic switch. You don't start to burn fat until about the fifth day of the program. Once you switch to a fat metabolism and your body adapts, you should feel energized. In fact, most people say they get a "rush" after four days. However, if symptoms continue, consult your health care practitioner.

► Is it dangerous to lose weight very quickly?

During Induction, you may experience rapid weight loss for the first time in your life. The initial drop in pounds is so dramatic because you lose a good amount of water weight in the first week. After four days or so, however, you will also begin to lose body fat. Young men and people who have a lot of weight to lose are more likely to lose weight faster at the start of the Atkins program.

Losing weight too fast is an issue of concern only if:

1. You're not eating enough, which could make you lose lean muscle mass. To lose only body fat, be sure to eat regular meals and take in adequate calories. If you aren't hungry at meal times, have a small snack with your supplements. Also, drink at least 64 ounces of water every day.
2. You feel sick, weak, dizzy or fatigued. If you lose pounds too fast, especially at the beginning of the program, you may be experiencing an extreme diuretic effect. This could deplete your body of water and also some electrolytes, which contain sodium, potassium,

calcium and magnesium. Signs of electrolyte
depletion are muscle cramps and heaviness in
your legs when climbing steps. You may need
to add more vegetables to your meals to slow
down weight loss and add a mineral supplement or drink mineral water or a low carb
sports drink to replace lost minerals.

But if you feel well and aren't starving yourself,
you're probably not losing weight too quickly. If you
have just a few pounds to lose, you might slow the
pace so that you can continue to learn good eating
habits before progressing through the phases to Lifetime Maintenance. Simply move to Ongoing Weight
Loss and increase your daily intake of carbohydrates
by 5 grams. However, if you still have a lot to lose and
you feel full of energy, simply relax and enjoy the fact
that you are dropping pounds easily! If you still don't
feel well, see your physician.

➤ **I have seen fat-burning products advertised to
   work synergistically with carbohydrate restricted diets. Are they in line with Atkins?**

Many products on the market claim to burn fat or
extra calories, increase energy or simply make you feel
great. These products rely on thermogenesis, the process by which your cells burn calories to manufacture
heat and produce energy. Preparations that contain
ephedra also produce such side effects as heartburn,
excessive stomach acid, increased blood cholesterol

and blood sugar, irregular heartbeat and elevated blood pressure. (Some products also blend aspirin with caffeine and ephedra to enhance thermogenesis.)

Ephedrine, ephedra's active compound, signals your adrenal glands to secrete adrenaline, which in turn encourages the breakdown of triglycerides and promotes the circulation of fatty acids in blood vessels, laying the groundwork for atherosclerosis. Ephedra can also increase the rate and force of one's heartbeat, an additive impact on the cardiovascular system that could cause a heart attack, and causes nervousness, irritability, even paranoia—especially in high doses. **We strongly advise against using ephedra in any form.**

Another compound promoted for controlled carb weight-loss efforts is phaseolamin, an extract of white kidney beans purported to act as a starch blocker, meaning it interferes with the absorption of carbs. It makes no sense to promote it to people already consuming low levels of carbohydrates. Moreover, reports of gastrointestinal complaints have been connected with its use. The presence of ingredients that inhibit trypsin, an enzyme produced by the pancreas, also is of concern. In animal studies, trypsin inhibitors have caused enlargement of the pancreas, but whether a similar effect occurs in humans is unknown.

► **Can patients with high uric acid (gout) safely do Atkins?**

If one has high uric acid or a history of gout, it is essential to maintain an adequate water intake at all times. Any rapid weight loss, including one resulting from doing Atkins, can exacerbate gout.

Doing Atkins can aggravate a pre-existing gout condition. Modification usually involves slowing down weight loss to fewer than two pounds a week and taking 300 milligrams of the prescription drug Allopurinol. If the uric acid level remains low, Allopurinol may be tapered down and stopped after one month—both should be done under a physician's care.

► **I've noticed some hair loss while I've been doing Atkins. Is this a result of my new eating habits?**

It is natural to go through periodic phases of shedding hair. But if this is an ongoing problem, make sure you're not restricting calories or skipping meals. Any low calorie weight-loss regimen may lower your metabolic rate, which can result in hair loss. Unlike calorie-restricted diets, Atkins is the least likely of any weight-loss program to contribute to hair loss because the higher caloric content prevents the body from behaving as though it is in a starvation mode. When that happens, your metabolism is lowered as a survival mechanism.

Alternatively, you might be low in some specific nutrients that could cause hair loss. Adding biotin, N-acetyl-cysteine (NAC), glutathione and lecithin to the diet has been found to help some people. If excessive hair loss occurs, see your doctor.

► **Why do I have terrible headaches while doing Atkins?**

Your headaches could be caused by a number of things related to the change in your eating patterns. The most common reason for headaches is caffeine withdrawal. If you were a big coffee or caffeinated soda drinker, this is very likely the cause of your headaches. Aspirin or ibuprofen may provide relief. Withdrawal from sugar and other carbohydrates also can cause headaches. If the cause is withdrawal, the headaches should stop after a few days.

Another common cause of headaches is food sensitivities. Are you now eating more of any food to which you might be sensitive? Foods and ingredients that frequently cause reactions include dairy products, nitrates (found in packaged processed meats, for example) and anything that's fermented, cured or smoked. If so, eliminate all the potential culprits by eating only natural, whole foods such as fresh meat, poultry, fish and vegetables for three or four days. After that, reintroduce one new food every 48 hours. Keep a food diary so you can document your reaction to each and determine which one might be causing the headaches.

Yet another possibility is that you are skipping meals. Doing so can trigger a drop in blood sugar that will often bring on a headache, especially if you wake with a headache or it is relieved by eating. You should be taking a multivitamin/mineral and essential oils supplement. Essential oils act as an anti-inflammatory agent, preventing headaches. (Headaches also may be caused by inflammation in the head or neck area or a nutrient deficiency.) Moreover, headaches can be one of the first signs of dehydration. So make sure you drink at least eight 8-ounce glasses of water each day. If none of these recommendations gives you relief, try seeing a chiropractor or osteopathic doctor to rule out a structural problem, such as poor posture or a pinched nerve.

► **Isn't doing Atkins bad for your heart?**

While you may have heard that a diet high in saturated fat causes heart disease or atherosclerosis (arteries clogged with cholesterol-laden plaque), it is actually a diet high in sugar and other refined carbohydrates *combined* with fat that is the real villain. Once you eliminate the bleached flour, sugar and other nutrient-empty carbohydrates from your diet, the fat you consume in meat or from other sources is burned for fuel (lipolysis) and is not converted into cholesterol or other harmful blood fats. Independent clinical studies indicate that cholesterol and triglyceride levels drop significantly on Atkins and levels of HDL ("good") cholesterol rise, often dramatically.

However, doing Atkins doesn't give you license to stuff yourself with well-marbled steaks or pounds of cheese at a sitting. The beneficial fats you should be consuming include the monounsaturated fats in olives and olive oil, nuts and nut oils, avocados and the all-important omega-3 fats found in fatty fish such as salmon, herring and tuna. Avoid trans fats (food labels refer to them as hydrogenated or partially hydrogenated oils). Found in packaged products such as crackers, bread, most margarines and peanut butters, and in commercially baked desserts and snacks, research has shown that these fats pose a serious risk of cardiac disease.

➤ **Since I started doing Atkins I have terrible leg cramps. How can I alleviate them?**

During the first week of Induction, in some people, Atkins has a strong diuretic effect. When you lose a large amount of water, as you do at the start of some weight-loss programs, you can lose electrolytes, the minerals sodium and potassium, and magnesium and calcium. This may result in leg cramps. To replace these vital nutrients, salt your food to taste and take a mineral supplement that includes calcium, magnesium and potassium.

➤ **While I am doing Atkins, which medical conditions should a physician monitor?**

A physician must monitor all medical conditions requiring prescriptions, and even some that don't, such as diet-controlled diabetes mellitus. This is necessary because following the Atkins Nutritional Approach™ and taking nutritional supplements improve many conditions, which can render prescribed drugs unnecessarily strong or lead to an overdose. Before starting Atkins (or any weight-loss regimen), everyone should get a complete history and physical from their physician, and repeat blood tests a few months after being on the program to track improvements in lipids.

► **Are there any medical conditions that can interfere with a person's ability to do Atkins?**

Before embarking on any weight-loss program you should see your physician for a checkup and have blood tests for lipid levels and routine chemistries, and possibly insulin levels, which can serve as baseline comparisons once you lose weight. **People with severe kidney disease should not do any phase of Atkins, unless prescribed by their physician. Also, pregnant women and nursing mothers may follow the Lifetime Maintenance phase but should not do any of the weight-loss phases of Atkins.** If you have a medical condition that requires you to follow specific protocols, work with your doctor to incorporate them into your diet.

► **Can you do Atkins if you have gallstones?**

Scientific evidence indicates that gallstones (responsible for more than 90 percent of gallbladder disease) form when fat intake is low. Gallbladders need to be kept active. Eating fat keeps the gallbladder working, which involves contraction for proper function; in fact, it will not contract without taking in fat. If the gallbladder isn't processing fat, bile salts crystallize into stones. People with existing gallstones may have trouble with high fat meals. If this is the case, you can follow a lower fat version of Atkins. Use fish, poultry, lean meats, low fat cheese (in moderation) and lots of vegetables. Stay away from creamy salad dressing; instead, use olive oil and vinegar or a mustard-based dressing. Eat nuts only in moderation. Don't fry foods, and use lean cuts of meat. Also avoid processed meats such as bacon and sausage. You may lose weight more slowly than people on the higher fat program do.

➤ **What medications interfere with or need to be adjusted while I am doing Atkins?**

You will need to stop taking any *unnecessary* over-the-counter medications, such as cough syrup or cough drops with added sugar. Many prescription medications may inhibit weight loss, among them birth control pills and hormone replacement therapy, steroids and anti-arthritis medications, beta-blockers and antidepressants. **Do not stop taking a medication or adjust the dosage without your doctor's approval.** Talk to your doctor to see if an alternative approach can be found.

There are also several categories of drugs that can cause adverse effects when taken while on a controlled carbohydrate eating plan. First are the diuretics, because reducing your carbohydrate intake alone can have a dramatic diuretic effect. Second, since Atkins is so effective at lowering high blood sugar, people who take insulin or oral diabetes medications that control blood sugar can end up with dangerously low blood sugar levels. You will need to be closely supervised in order to adjust your dosage, since the weight-loss phases of Atkins will naturally normalize your blood sugar levels. In combination with your pharmaceuticals, you could put yourself at risk for hypoglycemia. Third, Atkins has a strong blood-pressure-lowering effect and can easily convert blood-pressure medications into an overdose. If you are currently taking any of these medications, you will need your doctor's help to adjust your dosages. Be aware that overmedication may not occur immediately. Blood pressure may not fall until enough weight is lost. Monitoring your own blood pressure is essential so you can notify your doctor if your pressure drops too low.

► **Do aspirin and other pain relievers interfere with weight loss?**

Aspirin and Tylenol® do not interfere with weight loss, but some prescription drugs have that potential. Cortisone, for example, may actually cause you to gain weight. Although it is preferable to avoid the use of pharmaceuticals whenever possible, if you absolutely must take a pain reliever, discuss its side effects and possible impact on your weight with your physician.

► **Can I follow the Atkins Nutritional Approach™ while I'm pregnant?**

Weight loss by any method is not recommended while you are pregnant or breast-feeding, so the Atkins Lifetime Maintenance phase is best during this time.

As with all phases of Atkins, this entails building your eating program around protein, including meat, poultry and seafood, and healthy natural fats such as olive and flaxseed oil and avocados. Plenty of vegetables and one daily serving of fruit such as strawberries, blueberries or grapefruit are also included. Instead of hydrogenated oils, healthy fats, seeds and nuts are emphasized. As always, be sure to drink plenty of water.

The weight you gain over the full nine months will include the weight of the baby, placenta and fluid. It is advisable to control excessive gain caused by poor-quality foods such as sugar and refined flour products. It is especially important because of the risk of gestational diabetes.

► **Could an underactive thyroid be the reason it is so difficult for me to lose weight?**

Your thyroid gland's main function is to regulate the speed of your metabolism. If it is underactive—the medical word is "hypothyroid"—your slowed metabolism makes you more resistant to weight loss.

To find out whether you have hypothyroidism, your doctor will perform blood tests to evaluate your production of thyroid hormones T4 (also known as thyroxine) and T3 (your body converts T4 to T3), as well as another hormone called TSH (thyroid stimulating hormone). However, these clinical tests do not catch all cases. First think about whether you are experiencing any of the signs of an underactive thyroid. These symptoms include sensitivity to cold, weight gain, hair loss, fatigue and lethargy, depression, dry skin, chronic constipation, brittle nails, poor memory and elevated cholesterol levels.

➤ **My doctor has given me diuretics (water pills) because I retain water, especially before my period. How can I get off these pills?**

If water pills are prescribed simply for water retention and not for the treatment of heart disease or high blood pressure, you should be able to work with your doctor to wean yourself off. There are several nutrients that should allow you to safely stop these drugs. Supplements such as B-6, taurine and herbal preparations can be very useful. In addition, the use of a controlled carbohydrate way of eating has a strong diuretic effect, which helps to manage fluid problems. Of course, if these drugs are being used for the treatment of heart disease or high blood pressure, any changes must be made under medical supervision.

➤ **I have kidney stones. Will doing Atkins cause an attack?**

There is no evidence to indicate that people who do Atkins suffer a greater frequency of kidney stone attacks than people who follow another dietary regimen. If you have kidney stones, however, you *must* observe the rule about drinking eight or more glasses of water per day. Continue to see your doctor regularly so that he or she can monitor your condition.

▶ Doesn't doing Atkins increase the risk of osteoporosis by flushing calcium from the body?

Critics of the Atkins Nutritional Approach™ (ANA) have perpetuated the myth that controlling carbohydrate intake contributes to osteoporosis. They usually cite a series of short-term studies of people consuming a very high protein, low calorie diet that incorporates a protein powder for meal replacement, which showed increased calcium excretion in the urine. The studies looking at the ANA reported slightly increased calcium excretion in the urine that returned to normal after the first week. When more sophisticated tests looked at bone mass, there was no loss of bone. In fact, epidemiological studies of elderly women found that those who consumed the highest percentage of protein had better bone density than those who had lower protein consumption. It is important to understand that Atkins is not an excessively high protein regimen. The macronutrient breakout in the Induction phase is 60 percent fat, 30 percent protein and 10 percent carbohydrate. It should more appropriately be called a high fat regimen. As you progress through the phases, your percentage of fat naturally diminishes as your percentage of carbohydrate increases.

What is critical is that the typical American diet is very low in calcium. And even when you are eating calcium-rich foods, you should supplement with calcium, especially as you age, because progressive bone loss is inevitable. Most women take in less than half of what is needed to maintain healthy bones, and older women suffering broken bones as a result of osteoporosis is common. Men, too, can lose bone mass and develop osteoporosis. The Atkins approach includes foods high in calcium, including leafy green vegetables, cheese, sardines (with bones), seeds, nuts and soup stocks made with bones. We suggest that both men and women take a calcium supplement as well.

➤ **Every time I take supplements, I get sick to my stomach. What can I do?**

Don't stop taking your nutrients; instead, change the way you take them. Your nausea is almost certainly the result of an absorption problem. Supplements only occasionally cause side effects. When they do, symptoms tend to appear before absorption into the bloodstream. The side effects of drugs, on the other hand, usually appear only after the medications are surging through your arteries.

Be sure that you are taking your supplements with food. For some individuals, taking the supplements throughout the meal, which allows them to mix better with the food, works best. If that does not help, try the following:

The solution involves technique and timing. First, gather up all the supplements you would normally take during the day, put them in a food processor or blender and pulverize them. Divide the powder in half or into quarter portions. Take each portion over the course of the day, partway through each meal, not at the start. This is important, because you need some food in your stomach to stir the flow of gastric juices and better digest the nutrients.

You can mix the powdered supplements with anything you'd like—a bowl of soup or a glass of water, for example. We usually recommend adding the powder to Atkins Advantage™ Shake Mix. This technique works for most people. If it doesn't, try dividing the powder into even smaller portions.

There is also the possibility that a certain supplement brand is causing your nausea. Through a process of elimination, you can probably find out which one is the culprit. If you do identify a certain supplement, don't eliminate the nutrient(s) from your program; instead, switch to another manufacturer's product.

▶ Lipolysis and Ketosis

▶ What is ketosis?

Ketosis is really a shortening of the term lipolysis/ketosis. Lipolysis simply means that you're burning your fat stores and using them as the source of fuel they were meant to be. The by-products of burning fat are ketones, so ketosis is a secondary process of lipolysis. When your body releases ketones in your urine, it is chemical proof that you're consuming your own stored fat. And the more ketones you release, the more fat you have dissolved.

If you are restricting the amount of carbohydrate you eat, your body turns to fat as its alternative source of energy. In effect, lipolysis/ketosis has replaced the alternative of burning glucose for energy. Both are perfectly normal processes. People (and even some ill-informed doctors) often confuse ketosis, which is a perfectly normal metabolic process, with ketoacidosis, which is a life-threatening condition. The latter is the consequence of insulin-deficient subjects having out-of-control blood sugar levels, a condition that can also occur in alcoholics and people in a state of extreme starvation. Ketosis and ketoacidosis may sound vaguely alike, but the two conditions are virtually polar opposites and can always be distinguished from each other by the fact that the diabetic has been consuming excessive carbohydrates and has high blood sugar, in sharp contrast to the person who is doing Atkins.

► **Why does lipolysis/ketosis work?**

One of insulin's jobs is to convert excess carbohydrate into stores of body fat. In a normally functioning body, fatty acids and ketones are readily converted from fat tissue to fuel. But in overweight people, high insulin levels prevent this from happening.

Most obese people become so adept at releasing insulin that their blood is never really free of it and they're never able to use up their fat stores. By primarily burning fat instead of carbohydrates, lipolysis breaks the cycle of excess insulin and resultant stored fat. So by following a high fat, controlled carbohydrate regimen, you bypass the process of converting large amounts of carbohydrate into glucose. When your carbohydrate intake drops low enough to induce fat burning, abnormal insulin levels return to normal—perhaps for the first time in years or decades.

► How long does it usually take to get into ketosis?

The body can only store a two-day supply of glucose in the form of glycogen, so after two days of consuming no more than 20 grams of Net Carbs a day, most people go into lipolysis/ketosis. We recommend waiting four days before beginning to check your urine for ketones.

► What are lipolysis testing strips?

Lipolysis testing strips (LTS) measure the ketones—the markers that can indicate your body is in lipolysis and the secondary process of ketosis—in your urine. The strips will turn pink or purple, depending upon how many ketones are present. The more ketones you excrete, and therefore the greater degree of ketosis you are in, the darker the color. You don't have to use LTS, but doing so can be an extremely convenient aid to doing Atkins.

► What shade of purple should my lipolysis testing strips be? Will they show different levels at different times of day?

Because every person's metabolism is different, the sticks turn different shades of purple or pink for different people. And, yes, results vary depending upon the time of day, whether or not you exercise and what you last ate. It doesn't matter whether your strips turn a dark or light color. Some people never even get into ketosis but still lose weight easily. So don't worry about the exact level of ketosis shown on your test strips; what is more important is how your clothes are fitting, what the scale says and how you feel. Ketones can also be affected by hormone changes and can disappear before menses.

► How do I read lipolysis testing strips?

The package label shows various colors, but don't worry about the exact level of ketosis you will find on the strip. The strips are especially helpful in the Induction phase when you start doing Atkins. Later, as you move through the other phases and increase your carbohydrate intake, the strips are no longer needed. As long as you continue to lose weight gradually, lose inches, have your appetite under control, and experience none of your old symptoms, you are clearly burning fat. Moreover, in most cases, LTS will no longer turn pink or purple once you are taking in 50 or more grams of Net Carbs a day, so they are of no use above that level of carb intake.

► I am unable to get into ketosis even when I consume zero carbohydrates. What should I do?

Some people do not produce enough ketones for them to show up in their urine. If you are experiencing a reduction in your appetite and an improvement in well-being and are losing weight or your clothes are feeling looser, there is no need to do anything differently. Remember, the lipolysis testing strips (LTS) are tools; making them change color is not the sole object of following a controlled carb program.

If you are not losing weight, you either have a strong metabolic resistance to weight loss or you are consuming "hidden" carbohydrates in the form of sweetened salad dressing, breading, etc. In this case, follow Induction strictly for five days. If the LTS still haven't changed even slightly, make sure you are not consuming excess protein and measure your salads to make sure you are not eating too many veggies. Still no change? Try cutting out tomatoes and onions, which are relatively high on the glycemic index. You may also benefit from nutritional supplements such as L-carnitine, hydroxycitric acid (HCA), and chromium—all of which aid in hunger reduction or weight loss. You also may need to step up the frequency and intensity of your exercise sessions. **Note: Metabolic resistance can be increased by some medications. Also, some people with excessive insulin resistance are slower starters; patience is sometimes required.**

▶ **How long can I stay on Induction?**

The longer you consume no more than 20 grams of Net Carbs daily, the more body fat you will burn. Depending on how much weight you need to lose, you can safely continue with Induction as long as the following four conditions are met:

1. You have excess body fat to lose and are not within 10 pounds of your goal weight.
2. Your blood chemistries, lipid values, blood pressure or blood sugar levels continue to improve or remain stable and within normal limits.
3. You feel well and are experiencing a high energy level, normal sleep patterns and stable moods.
4. You are not bored. Boredom could lead to cheating and undermine your efforts.

However, it is important to understand the entire Atkins Nutritional Approach™. The ultimate goal of the program is to advance from the Induction phase through Ongoing Weight Loss and Pre-Maintenance, culminating in Lifetime Maintenance, which should become your permanent way of eating. By following these steps, you can find your Critical Carbohydrate Level for Losing (CCLL), also known as your carbohydrate threshold for losing, and ultimately your Atkins Carbohydrate Equilibrium (ACE), also known as your carbohydrate threshold for maintaining. Segueing from one phase to another will help you maintain a healthy weight, feel good and decrease your risk factors for chronic diseases such as heart disease, hypertension and diabetes.

That being said, if you have a great deal of weight to lose, you can certainly stay on Induction for six months or even more. When you switch to Ongoing Weight Loss, your rate of loss will naturally diminish. On the other hand, if you have a modest weight loss goal, say 20 pounds, and lose the first pounds rapidly, it is important to move through the more liberal phases so you can establish the good eating habits that will become part of your ongoing lifestyle and end a pattern of yo-yo dieting.

➤ **Doesn't ketosis lead to loss of muscle mass?**

The notion that the Atkins Nutritional Approach™— high in protein, which builds muscle, and fat, which is used for energy—will force your body to break down muscle is incorrect. Only individuals on very low calorie diets can lose muscle mass, because they have an inadequate protein intake. Atkins, however, is not calorie restricted (this isn't an invitation for gorging, but a recommendation to eat until you are no longer hungry) and the high protein intake offsets any possible loss of body mass.

➤ **Nutritional Supplements**

➤ **What is the advantage of taking Atkins supplements instead of other brands?**

Atkins brand supplements use only high-quality ingredients. We do not use cheap fillers and additives such as plastics, wax, and artificial colors and flavors.

There are also no hydrogenated oils, digestive yeast, corn, wheat, salt, sugar, starch or gluten in Atkins supplements. Our products have also been formulated based on more than 30 years of observations and experience at Dr. Atkins' medical practice.

▶ Phases of the Atkins Nutritional Approach™

▶ How do I know when to move from one phase of Atkins to the next?

You are ready to leave Induction after a minimum of two weeks. If you have a lot of weight to lose, you can stay on Induction until at least the first 30 percent of your weight is lost. Or you may be bored with the options available on Induction and want to trade a slow-down in the progress of your weight loss in return for eating a wider variety of foods. The next phase is called Ongoing Weight Loss (OWL), when each week you increase your daily Net Carb intake by 5 grams in the form of nutrient-dense foods, such as vegetables, seeds and nuts, and low-glycemic fruits such as berries. So the first week on OWL, you go from 20 to 25 grams per day; the following week you would move to 30 grams per day and so on. Change the increments on a weekly basis until your weight loss slows to one to two pounds each week. Slowly increasing your carb intake allows your body to continue to use its fat stores for fuel.

When you are within 5 or 10 pounds of your target weight, it is time to move to Pre-Maintenance. You will now be broadening your range of foods while learning what you can eat without regaining weight, adding 10 grams of daily Net Carbs in weekly increments. So long as you continue to lose weight at a slow, almost imperceptible rate, you can begin to add starchy vegetables and whole grains, such as brown rice or whole-wheat bread. However, if adding these foods results in cravings or makes you gain weight, you should stop eating them immediately.

After you have maintained your weight for four weeks, you will have transitioned to the phase called Lifetime Maintenance, where you are eating a whole-foods diet. On rare occasions, you may be able to indulge in a slice of cake or another dessert, but in general you will continue to avoid products full of sugar and bleached flour to maintain your weight.

➤ **Can I eat Atkins Advantage™ Bars during the Induction phase?**

An Advantage bar can serve as either a snack or an *occasional* meal replacement. Feel free to eat them during Induction as long as you continue to lose weight. (We generally recommend no more than one bar or shake a day during the first two weeks of Induction.) But keep in mind that neither the Atkins shakes nor the bars were formulated to be total meal replacements. Atkins does not recommend the use of meal replacements for more than one meal a day; instead, it is important to eat whole, unprocessed foods and to learn wholesome eating habits.

► **Why can't I eat Atkins Endulge™ Bars during Induction?**

It is prudent to avoid Endulge products during the first two weeks of Induction, to be sure that cravings for sweets are under control and your body is firmly in the fat-burning metabolism.

► **I'm used to counting calories. How many am I allowed on Induction?**

The Atkins Nutritional Approach™ counts grams of carbohydrates instead of calories. During Induction, you are allowed 20 grams of Net Carbs a day. When you progress to Ongoing Weight Loss, you gradually add carbohydrates in 5-gram increments per week as you move toward Pre-Maintenance, and finally in 10-gram increments per week as you approach the Lifetime Maintenance phase. Although you do not need to count calories, it is certainly possible to consume too many calories even if your carb intake is on target. If you are losing weight, there is no need to concern yourself with counting calories. However, if you are unable to lose weight or actually regain weight lost, one possibility is that you are taking in more calories than you expend through exercise, thermogenesis (the body's own heat production) and other metabolic functions. Excess protein intake can be converted to glucose. When there is more glucose present there is less fat burning. We recommend that you eat until satisfied, not stuffed.

Research has shown that on a controlled carbohydrate program, more calories are burned than on a low fat, high carbohydrate diet, so there is a certain metabolic advantage to the controlled carb approach. But understand that this does not give you a license to gorge.

If you are used to counting calories and are more comfortable with such an approach, the general rule of thumb is to multiply your present weight by 10 to 12 to get the daily caloric range at which you would lose weight. For example, a 150-pound woman who consumes 1,500 to 1,800 calories daily should continue to lose weight.

The real goal of the Atkins program is to learn eating habits that will enable you to permanently maintain a healthy weight and lifestyle. This includes changing old habits such as overeating that contributed to your original weight problem.

➤ **You don't use the term "The Atkins Diet" anymore. Why not?**

The word "diet" has several meanings, the most basic one referring to the food we regularly eat. But in our culture, the word has become intertwined with weight loss and implies a limited period during which intake is restricted in order to lose weight. No matter how successful they may be in losing weight, most people go off their "diet" and return to their normal way of eating—and then regain the weight they have lost.

In contrast, the Atkins Nutritional Approach™ refers to a lifestyle and four graduated phases that encompass weight loss and weight maintenance as well as overall health and well-being and the reduction of risk factors for heart disease, diabetes and other illnesses. Depending upon your weight and health, you can personalize Atkins to suit your individual needs and move from one phase of the program to another as your needs change. Atkins is more than a diet—it is a healthful approach to eating that will serve you for the rest of your life.

► **What is carb creep and how can I avoid it?**

When you start adding back carbohydrates as you move from Induction into the progressively less restrictive phases of Atkins, some people begin to lose track of how many grams of Net Carbs they're eating. If that happens, you are likely to stop weight loss or regain the pounds you've already lost. That is why it is very important to increase your daily carb intake by only 5 grams each week and to introduce only one new food at a time. That way, you'll also immediately notice if a new food is causing you to experience cravings that lead to overeating. Another way to stay in control is to keep a food diary so you can spot troublesome foods before they set up a pattern of cravings and gorging. For example, if you find that after eating nuts you are hungry again in a few hours, cut out the nuts and see if the hunger disappears.

▶ **After months of doing Atkins, I started cheating. What's the best way to get back on plan?**

When someone "cheats," they often experience carbohydrate cravings caused by unstable blood sugar levels. The first thing you need to do is go back on Induction for a week or so to get your blood sugar level under control. When you are no longer craving foods high in carbohydrates and your energy level feels stable, you can move beyond Induction again. Pay careful attention to what happened that led you to "fall off the wagon" and make sure not to let it happen again. Falling off the wagon can be useful, if you learn from the experience. What you learn can help to limit future episodes and you will have one more tool to assist in Lifetime Maintenance. But don't fall into the trap of being too strict and denying yourself completely; this could lead to more cheating. Giving yourself an occasional treat—within your carbohydrate threshold—is part of the Atkins approach.

▶ **What is the highest level of carbohydrate consumption per day recommended for Lifetime Maintenance?**

The important concept to understand in order to maintain your weight is what we call the Atkins Carbohydrate Equilibrium (ACE), the number of grams of Net Carbs at which you neither gain nor lose weight. You should find the highest level of carbohydrate consumption that won't allow you to regain weight or cause hunger and cravings. Depending upon age, activity level, hormonal status, and genetics, each person has an individual ACE, and a bit of trial and error may be required for you to find yours.

➤ Slow Weight Loss and Plateaus

➤ **Could eating Atkins Advantage™ Bars be impeding my weight loss?**

This varies by individual. If you are doing everything right but are not losing weight, try omitting the bars until weight loss resumes. Alternatively, you could exercise more to burn the extra calories or try eating only half a bar. Remember, each bar contains approximately 220 calories and these calories could be affecting your overall weight loss. The controlled carb way of eating has an advantage over low fat diets in that you can take in more calories and still lose more weight; but don't regard this as a license to overeat.

➤ **My sister and I are both doing Atkins, but she is losing weight much more quickly than I am. What's my problem?**

First, assuming that you are doing Atkins properly, recognize that there may not be a problem at all. Different people will respond to Atkins differently; some consistently lose weight while others do so in stages.

Don't compare yourself to others and become overly concerned with short-term results. Certain medications, activity level, hormonal status and age can cause differences in weight loss. Also, make sure your expectations of weight loss are realistic. Atkins is designed to lead you to your natural weight. For many people, that may still be more than they wish to weigh. We strongly recommend that you manage your expectations in a real and healthy way.

Second, remember that success on Atkins is measured by more than just the scale. Consider the following questions and think about how they apply to your experience doing Atkins:

- Are you experiencing more energy and vitality throughout the day?
- Are your clothes fitting you better?
- Are you experiencing less between-meal cravings and hunger?
- Have your blood lipid tests improved?
- Are you losing weight, but at a slow pace?
- Have you lost inches?

If you answered "yes" to any of the above, then you have the right plan for the rest of your life. Continue to stick with it, modifying it as you go along to make it work for you, and you will continue to see suitable health-enhancing results.

➤ Sweeteners

➤ **What kinds of sweeteners do you recommend?**

A main goal of the Atkins Nutritional Approach™ is to stabilize blood sugar (glucose) and insulin levels through the restriction of carbohydrates. Sugar is a carbohydrate, so it is strictly limited. Controlling carbs naturally curbs sugar cravings. However, if you still crave sweets, we suggest you use a sugar substitute. The prudent, moderate use of artificial sweeteners is usually acceptable. But be aware that not all sugar substitutes are created equal. We recommend specific sweeteners that are safe and will not interfere with weight loss. Some people experience negative reactions to certain sweeteners, and the risk increases with the amount used. With all artificial sweeteners, the less used, the better.

Our preference is for sucralose, marketed under the name Splenda®. Derived from sugar, it is non-caloric, contains less than 1 gram of carbs and doesn't raise blood sugar. It has been used in Canada since 1991 and has been thoroughly tested for safety and efficacy. Sucralose is approximately 600 times sweeter than sugar. It is inert in the body's digestive system, quickly passing through without accumulating in tissues. In addition, it does not lose its sweetness when heated, so it can be used in cooking and baking.

In 1998, the Food and Drug Administration (FDA) approved sucralose for sale in the United States after reviewing more than 100 studies conducted during the previous 20 years.

If Splenda® is not available, saccharin is the next best thing. The FDA recently removed saccharin from its list of carcinogens, basing its decision upon a thorough review of the medical literature and the National Institute of Environmental Health Sciences' statement that "there is no clear association between saccharin and human cancer." It can be safely consumed in moderate amounts—no more than three packets a day. Sugar poses a greater threat to good health than saccharin does. Saccharin is marketed as Sweet 'N Low®.

Acesulfame potassium, also known as acesulfame-K, another non-caloric sweetener, is approximately 200 times sweeter than sugar. Because it cannot be metabolized, it passes through the body without elevating blood sugar. The FDA has authorized the use of acesulfame-K after evaluating numerous studies and determining its safety. It is sold under the brand name Sunett™.

Avoid natural sweeteners such as fructose, lactose or maltose.

▶ **What are sugar alcohols?**

While most carbohydrates—sugar is the best example—are digested and turned into blood sugar, other carbs behave differently. Some are digested by your body but not turned into glucose and some carbs—such as fiber—are not digested at all, and pass through your body as waste. Sugar alcohols, such as maltitol, are often used as sweeteners in low carb products because they have a minimal impact on blood sugar.

► **How do I know how much sugar substitute to use when adapting recipes?**

Generally, one packet of any sugar substitute has the sweetening power of two teaspoons of sugar. Splenda®, which is a combination of sucralose and maltodextrin, comes in packets ideal for sweetening decaf tea or decaf coffee. It also comes in a granulated form, which can be substituted for sugar, measure for measure. A 3.8-ounce box is equivalent in sweetening ability to two pounds of sugar. (Splenda® is lighter than sugar.) Simply substitute it for sugar in your favorite recipes. Keep in mind that all sugar substitutes contain about 0.9 gram of carbohydrate, which you should count as 1 gram. Be sure to account for the amount you use in recipes in your daily carb count.

► **I used artificial sweetener in a recipe and the finished product tasted bitter. What did I do wrong?**

Certain artificial sweeteners lose their effect when heated. This is especially true of aspartame. Try switching to a heatproof sweetener, such as Splenda®.

► Weight Management

► **I'm of normal weight but want to do Atkins for health reasons. Can I restrict carbohydrates without losing weight?**

The Atkins Nutritional Approach™ is recommended for much more than weight loss. Almost everyone will experience health benefits by controlling carbohydrates. The average American eats about 300 grams of carbohydrates a day, half of it as sugar.

Here's how to adapt Atkins to your needs. Start with the Ongoing Weight Loss phase, where in addition to protein, fats and vegetables, you will be eating seeds, nuts and berries. If you find you are losing weight, add higher carb vegetables such as yams, turnips and winter squash. There are also certain low-glycemic legumes such as lentils and soybeans and low-glycemic fruits such as melon and apricots that you may be able to incorporate. Finally, add whole grains. While consuming your normal amount of protein, add as much of these foods as you wish, so long as you maintain your normal weight. Everyone, however slim, should avoid empty carbs in the form of refined bleached flour or sugar, including most processed foods. Similarly, no matter what your weight, you should supplement your diet with vitamins, minerals and essential fatty acids and adhere to a regular exercise program.

► Women's Health

► Will the Atkins Nutritional Approach™ interfere with the efficacy of birth control pills or will the pills hinder success on Atkins?

There has been no research to evaluate the effect of any weight-loss program on the efficacy of oral contraceptives. However, because birth control pills contain estrogen, they may impact your ability to lose weight on Atkins. Estrogen causes more fat to be stored in your tissues rather than being burned as energy. This increases insulin resistance, making weight loss more difficult. Estrogen also lowers thyroid function, which is necessary to keep your metabolism at an appropriate active level. If you have no choice but to take birth control pills, be prepared for the fact that your carbohydrate threshold may be lower than it would be otherwise, requiring you to be extra vigilant about your carb intake.

► I have polycystic ovarian syndrome (PCOS). Can doing Atkins help?

Polycystic ovarian syndrome is a hormonal imbalance that causes painful, irregular menstruation, infertility, weight gain, excess body hair, and even symptoms of diabetes. It is likely that abnormal insulin production and/or insulin resistance play a role in the cause of PCOS. A controlled carbohydrate program has been shown to help keep PCOS symptoms under control and prevent long-term complications.

► Glossary

A

Absorption: A process by which food molecules enter cells after digestion.

Allergic reaction (allergy): A condition caused by a response of the body's immune system to what it identifies as a foreign substance.

Amino acids: A large group of organic compounds that are the end product of protein metabolism, in turn used by the body to rebuild protein. Many amino acids are necessary to maintain life.

Antidepressant: A substance or a measure that prevents or relieves the debilitating effects of depression.

Antihistamine: A pharmaceutical, over-the-counter drug or natural agent that opposes the action of histamine, which is released by the body in response to an allergic reaction, causing dilated capillaries, decreased blood pressure, increased gastric secretion and constriction of bronchial tubes.

Antioxidant: A chemical or other agent that inhibits or retards oxidation, whose by-products can cause premature aging, cancer, heart disease, arthritis and other diseases. Antioxidants are known to reverse, prevent or limit free-radical damage.

Arthritis: An inflammatory joint condition characterized by pain, swelling, heat, redness and restricted movement. There are various types of arthritis, including rheumatoid arthritis and osteoarthritis. Approximately 350 million people worldwide have arthritis.

Atherosclerosis: The slow, progressive buildup of hardened deposits called plaques on the inner walls of arteries, cutting down on the flow of oxygen-rich blood and nutrients to the heart. It is a major cause of coronary artery (heart) disease. Plaques are deposits of fat, cholesterol, calcium and other cellular sludge carried in the blood. Atherosclerosis is also typically a by-product of poor health habits. When the level of cholesterol in the blood is high, there's a greater chance that it will be deposited on artery walls. High blood pressure, high insulin levels, smoking, obesity and physical inactivity also contribute to the risk of atherosclerosis, and thus, coronary artery disease. Some research also suggests that certain types of bacteria, such as *Chlamydia pneumoniae,* may play a role in narrowing coronary arteries. Atherosclerosis also can occur in the arteries that carry blood to the brain, increasing the risk of a stroke.

Atkins Carbohydrate Equilibrium: Also known as ACE, the number of grams of Net Carbs you can eat without gaining or losing weight.

B

Blood chemistry: A measure of various substances, including electrolytes, protein and glucose, and the number of red and white blood cells per cubic millimeter of blood. A complete blood count is one of the most routinely performed tests in a clinical laboratory, as well as one of the most valuable screening and diagnostic techniques to help evaluate health status.

Blood lipid profile: Results of blood tests that reveal a person's total cholesterol, triglycerides and various lipoproteins. This test must be done with an overnight fast for accurate results. Also called a lipoprotein profile.

Blood pressure: The amount of force exerted against the blood vessels to push blood to and from the heart. Every time the heart contracts or beats (systolic), blood pressure increases. When the heart relaxes between beats (diastolic), the pressure decreases. Blood pressure can fluctuate considerably, depending on factors such as diet and stress. Generally, healthy systolic values are under 120 and diastolic values are below 80; expressed as 120 over 80.

Blood sugar: The level of glucose detected in the bloodstream as determined by blood tests. Typically, normal blood glucose levels are between 70 and 109 mg/dL.

Body mass index (BMI): A measurement of a person's weight in relation to his or her height. The value is associated with body fat and health risks. The formula for calculating your BMI is BMI = [Weight in pounds ÷ Height in inches ÷ Height in inches] × 703. Fractions and ounces must be entered as decimal values. The metric formula is

BMI = Body Weight(kg)/height(m)^2. A BMI between 19 and 24 is considered healthy; between 25 and 29.9 is considered overweight; more than 30 is considered obese.

C

Caffeine: A natural stimulant found in many common foods and beverages, including coffee, tea, cola drinks and chocolate. It may enhance exercise endurance by stimulating fatty acid release, but also causes fluid loss. Consuming too much caffeine can lead to headaches, trembling, rapid heart rate and other undesirable side effects. Excessive caffeine can also cause unstable blood sugar and therefore lead to binge eating.

Calcium: A mineral that builds and maintains bones and teeth, calcium is also essential for blood clotting and nerve transmission. There are various forms of calcium that are available in supplement form, however, calcium hydroxyapatite, orotate and citrate are those most readily absorbed.

Calorie: A unit by which energy is measured. Food energy is actually measured in kilocalories (1,000 calories = 1 kilocalorie), which is abbreviated as kcalories or kcal.

Cancer: An abnormal and uncontrolled growth of cells, it is not a single disease, but a term that encompasses more than 100 different and distinctive diseases. Cancer may be benign (meaning it does not spread to other parts of the body and is not life-threatening) or malignant (when cells invade and damage nearby tissues and organs and can spread to different areas of the body, a process called metastasis).

Carbohydrate: One of the nutrients that supply calories to the body. Compounds composed of carbon, oxygen and hydrogen arranged as monosaccharides (simple sugars) or multiples of monosaccharides (polysaccharides). Sources include grains, fruits, vegetables, nuts, legumes and other plant foods. When completely broken down in the body, a gram of carbohydrate yields about four calories.

Cardiac risk: The chance of having a disease related to the heart. Blood measurement of total cholesterol, triglycerides, HDL and LDL will be calculated to determine risk ratio as being high or low. Other risk factors include smoking, obesity, diabetes, stress, physical inactivity, increasing age and family history.

Cholesterol: Also known as serum cholesterol. A soft waxy substance present in all parts of the body including the nervous system, skin, muscle, liver, intestines and heart. It is made by the body and obtained from fatty substances in the diet. Cholesterol is manufactured in the liver for normal body functions, including the production of hormones, bile and vitamin D. It is transported in the blood for use by all parts of the body.

Cold-pressed oil: Oil that has been extracted by squeezing seeds in a press. Also known as "expeller-pressed" oil. This method differs from the standard, chemically induced method in which heat and hexane gas are used to extract oil. Using the cold-pressed method to extract oil ensures that it has no hexane molecules and no poisonous trans fatty acids.

Complex carbohydrates: Polysaccharides composed of straight or branched chains of monosaccharides (simple sugars).

Constipation: The condition of having infrequent or difficult bowel movements.

Controlled carbohydrate diet: A lifestyle that includes limiting the intake of carbohydrate to lose and maintain weight by emphasizing whole, nutrient-dense foods.

Coronary heart disease: A general term used to describe diseases affecting the heart or blood vessels, including but not limited to atherosclerosis, coronary artery disease, arrhythmia, heart failure, hypertension, endocarditis and congenital heart disease.

Critical carbohydrate level for losing (CCLL): The level of carbohydrate intake that will allow an overweight individual to lose weight doing Atkins. The number of daily grams of Net Carbs at which weight loss occurs.

D

Diabetes: A disorder characterized by high fasting blood sugar levels (126 mg/dL and higher) and the inability of the body to transport glucose to cells. See **Type 1 diabetes** and **Type 2 diabetes**.

Diastolic blood pressure: The point of least blood pressure, when the heart dilates between each heartbeat. It is the lower number in a blood pressure reading, expressed as the bottom part, or denominator, of the fraction. When you say your blood pressure is 110 over 70, 70 is the diastolic blood pressure.

Dietary cholesterol: Chemically, a compound composed of carbon, hydrogen and oxygen atoms arranged in rings. It is found only in animal foods such as meat, eggs and dairy products, as well as shellfish. In the body, dietary cholesterol serves as a structural component of cell membranes and contributes to other functions. It had a bad rap for giving people high serum (blood) cholesterol levels until researchers determined that the liver contributes much more cholesterol to the body's total count than does diet.

Dietary fiber: Plant cell walls and other non-nutritive residues that are not digested are generally called dietary fiber. Fibers include cellulose, pectins, gums, lignans, cutins and tannins.

Digestion: The process of breaking down food particles into molecules small enough to be absorbed by cells.

Diuretic: Any process or factor that increases urine output. Diuretic drugs are prescribed for the treatment of edema (the accumulation of excess fluids in the tissues of the body), which may be the result of underlying disease of the kidneys, liver, lungs or heart (e.g., congestive heart failure). Fluid retention also can be the result of a high-salt diet, excessive insulin production, hormone imbalances or food allergies. Diuretics are also used to treat high blood pressure and glaucoma. They act on the kidneys, modifying the absorption and excretion of water and electrolytes such as sodium and potassium.

Diverticulosis: A condition characterized by small pouches (diverticula) that form in the wall of the large intestine. When the pouches become infected or inflamed, the condition is called diverticulitis, which produces symptoms such as abdominal pain, nausea, vomiting, constipation or diarrhea, fever and frequent urination. If early symptoms are ignored, perforation of the colon and peritonitis can occur. Consuming adequate amounts of fiber to ensure bowel regularity is the best prescription against developing diverticulosis.

E

Eczema: Also known as atopic dermatitis, eczema is a chronic skin condition whose cause is unknown.

Electrolytes: Salts such as sodium, calcium, potassium, chlorine, magnesium and bicarbonate in blood, tissue and other cells, electrolytes consist of various chemicals that can carry electric charges. Proper quantities and balance of electrolytes are essential to normal metabolism and function. Diuretics can cause loss of electrolytes, resulting in leg cramps and other symptoms.

Enzyme: A protein that acts as a catalyst for a biological reaction. For example, digestive enzymes facilitate the breakdown of food in digestion.

Essential amino acids: Nine amino acids that the human body cannot synthesize and must be obtained from food.

Essential fat: The kind of fat deemed absolutely necessary for the body to function properly but which cannot be produced by the body. Examples include the omega-3 and omega-6 fatty acids.

Essential fatty acids: Polyunsaturated acids that are essential in the diet, they are commonly called EFAs and include linolenic (omega-3) and linoleic acid (omega-6). Sources of EFAs are seeds (including flaxseed), oils (safflower, sunflower, corn) and deep-sea fish. They are necessary for normal functioning of the endocrine and reproductive systems and for breaking up cholesterol deposits on arterial walls. EFAs play an important role in fat transport and metabolism and in maintaining the function and integrity of cellular membranes. A deficiency in EFAs causes changes in cell structure and enzyme function, decreased rate of growth, brittle and dull hair, nail problems, dandruff, allergic conditions and skin problems. Supplementation with EFAs has proven useful in treating high cholesterol, neurological disorders and other medical conditions. It also assists in weight loss.

Estrogens: A class of female sex hormones produced by the ovaries that bring about sexual maturation at puberty and maintain reproductive functions.

Excretion: The removal of metabolic wastes from the body.

F

Fat: A water-insoluble solid or semisolid compound that is one of the three sources of macronutrients (supplying calories) in food and essential for life. Fat insulates the body—ensuring temperature maintenance—supplies fatty acids and carries the fat-soluble vitamins A, D, E and K. When completely broken down in the body, a gram of fat yields about 9 calories. Total fat refers to the sum of saturated, monounsaturated and polyunsaturated fats in food.

Fat-producing hormone: See **insulin**.

Fatty acids: An acid originating from fats such as oleic, stearic and palmitic acid.

Fiber: See **dietary fiber**.

Food allergy: See **allergic reaction.**

Food intolerance: An adverse reaction to foods that does not involve the immune system, and is therefore less severe than a food allergy. A common example is lactose intolerance, caused by the inability to digest the lactose (milk sugar) found in dairy products.

Fructose: A simple sugar found in fruit, honey, corn and saps. It has the same chemical formula as glucose and therefore may be used as a source of energy like glucose or converted to glycogen and stored in the body.

G

Gallbladder: A hollow, pear-shaped organ located beneath the liver, it stores and concentrates bile, which emulsifies fat.

Gallstones: Stones in the gallbladder that vary in size from a small seed to that of a lemon and can slow or obstruct the flow of bile and can result in gallbladder disease.

Glucose: A form of simple sugar also known as blood sugar or dextrose.

Glycemic index (GI): A quick way to understand the relative impact that carbohydrates from a particular food have on your blood sugar compared to the effect after eating a similar amount of pure glucose, which enters your bloodstream almost immediately. In general, the lower a food is on the GI, the less glucose it will deliver to your bloodstream and therefore the less insulin your pancreas must produce to transport the glucose to your cells. And the less insulin you produce, the less likely it is that your body is going to store fat. The GI does not take into account the average size of a portion.

Glycerine: Also known as glycerol or glycerin, this sugar alcohol is a thick liquid used by food manufacturers to improve taste, add moisture and impart sweetness. Glycerine is classed as a carbohydrate, but does not impact on blood sugar levels the way such carbohydrates as cane sugar does. Consequently, it can be used as a replacement for cane sugar; glycerine is 0.6 times as sweet as cane sugar. Chemically, it is a three-carbon molecule with three hydroxyl groups, and is one of the most common alcohols found in human metabolism. It is also found naturally in animal and plant products and is the backbone of triglycerides (fats) and phospholipids.

Glycogen: A complex sugar composed of glucose, it is manufactured and stored in the liver and muscles and held ready for release to other parts of the body.

Glycolysis: The energy-yielding process of converting glucose to pyruvic and lactic acids.

Gout: A type of arthritis or inflammation of a joint caused by excess uric acid in the blood. Attacks occur suddenly and are characterized by severe pain and tenderness. The big toe is a frequent site. In the past, gout was associated with obese old men who overindulged in rich foods. But today it's recognized that anyone can develop gout. In fact, gout is a painful problem for more than two million Americans. Men are more likely to get gout, but women become increasingly susceptible to it after menopause.

H

HDL (high-density lipoprotein): Considered the "good" cholesterol, HDL is actually a carrier molecule that transports cholesterol in the blood. HDL is responsible for returning cholesterol and triglycerides (fats) from the cells and the vessels to the liver. A high HDL blood level is associated with a lowered risk of heart attack.

HDL/LDL ratio: The ratio of high-density lipoprotein to low-density lipoprotein cholesterol levels in the blood.

Heart disease: Also known as coronary artery disease, this is any one of the abnormal conditions that may clog the heart's arteries with a buildup of plaque from cholesterol, calcium or mechanical trauma. The buildup produces various pathologic effects, especially reduced flow of oxygen and nutrients to the myocardium (the heart muscle). Coronary atherosclerosis, one type of coronary artery disease, is the leading cause of death in the Western world.

High blood pressure: Also known as hypertension, high or elevated blood pressure is a major risk factor for heart attack or stroke. Blood pressure represents the resistance produced each time the heart beats and sends blood flowing through the arteries. The top reading of the pressure exerted by this contraction is called systolic pressure. Between beats, the heart relaxes and blood pressure drops. The lower reading is referred to as diastolic pressure. It is estimated that 24 percent of all American adults (about 43 million people) have high blood pressure.

High blood sugar: See **hyperglycemia**.

Hormonal cycles: A complex monthly balance of hormones that affect menstruation and ovulation. The hypothalamus, pituitary gland, estrogen, progesterone, luteinizing hormone and follicle-stimulating hormone are all part of the hormonal cycle.

Hydrogenated oil: A man-made product (unsaturated fat to which a hydrogen molecule is added) causing an oil to become more solid at room temperature. Considered a saturated fat, it is used by the food industry to prolong the shelf life of many processed foods, such as sliced bread, margarine, vegetable shortenings, soups, chips, crackers, cookies, pastries and even some pasta and rice mixes.

Hyperglycemia: A condition in which there is a greater than normal amount of glucose in the blood, and which can lead to serious conditions such as Type 2 diabetes.

Hyperinsulinemia: A condition in which the pancreas releases excess amounts of insulin into the blood, usually in an effort to control high blood sugar. It may be a precursor to diabetes, is an independent risk factor for heart disease and is associated with many medical conditions such as syndrome X, or metabolic syndrome, and high blood pressure. Characteristics of hyperinsulinemia include sodium retention, thickening of artery walls causing constriction and can contribute to certain cancers.

Hyperinsulinism: The body's reaction to an excessive amount of carbohydrate consumption, which raises blood sugar and, in turn, produces high insulin levels.

Hypertension: See **high blood pressure**.

Hypoglycemia: A condition in which there is a lower than normal amount of glucose in the blood. This can happen when glucose is used up too rapidly, glucose is released into the bloodstream more slowly than is needed by the body or when excessive insulin (a hormone secreted by the pancreas in response to increased glucose levels in the blood) is released into the bloodstream. Hypoglycemia is relatively common in prediabetes.

Hypothyroidism: A condition of decreased activity of the thyroid gland, which may cause a variety of symptoms. The body's normal rate of functioning slows, causing

mental and physical sluggishness, lethargy, water retention, constipation, depression, high cholesterol, dry skin,
brittle nails and hair loss.

I

Induction: The initial phase of the Atkins Nutritional Ap-
proach™, which lasts a minimum of two weeks. During
this time, it is recommended that Net Carb consumption
not exceed 20 grams a day, in order to trigger lipolysis/
ketosis, in which the body burns its own fat for energy.
After this phase, more grams of carbohydrate and a
broader array of foods are gradually introduced, deliberately slowing the pace of weight loss.

Insulin: A naturally occurring hormone secreted by the pancreas that helps transport glucose into muscle cells and
other tissue, where it is stored for energy use. Insulin is
also known as the fat-producing hormone.

Insulin resistance: Reduced sensitivity of the body to insulin's effect on blood sugar. When there is ongoing intake of excessive carbohydrates, there is a corresponding
flow of insulin responses; over time, the receptors become less sensitive and can no longer transport the excess
glucose, resulting in fat buildup, insulin resistance and,
ultimately, Type 2 diabetes.

K

Ketoacidosis: A state in which there is an abnormal accumulation of ketones, which changes the body's PH to
acidic. This usually occurs in diabetics whose blood
sugar is out of control, alcoholics and people in a state of

starvation. Ketoacidosis is not to be confused with keto-sis, which is a perfectly normal function of burning fat for energy.

Ketone: The normal products of fat metabolism, when there is not sufficient carbohydrate as a source of energy. For people who are restricting their intake of carbohydrates, ketone presence in the urine indicates achievement of a fat-burning phase that will result in weight loss. Also known as ketone bodies.

Ketosis: Short for benign dietary ketosis, or BDK, this is a biological process that results when sufficient glucose as a source of energy is not available from dietary carbohydrate and the body switches to primarily using fat. Fatty acids are released into the bloodstream, then converted to ketones, which are used by muscles, the brain and other organs. Excess ketones are excreted in urine.

Kidneys: The pair of organs that regulate blood chemistry and remove water and metabolic wastes from the blood.

L

Lactose: A disaccharide composed of glucose and galactose; commonly known as milk sugar.

LDL (low-density lipoprotein): LDL is a carrier molecule that transports cholesterol and triglycerides in the blood from the liver to the body's cells. A high level of LDL is associated with a high risk of heart attack because it indicates there is too much artery-clogging cholesterol in the blood. Although long considered the "bad" cholesterol, recent research indicates that some sub-fractions of LDL are actually heart protective.

Lifetime Maintenance: In the Atkins Nutritional Approach™, Lifetime Maintenance is the final phase in which desired weight loss has been attained and is sustained by ascertaining the individual's Atkins Carbohydrate Equilibrium (ACE).

Lipid: A group of organic compounds that includes fats and oils. Examples of fatty substances in the blood include cholesterol, free fatty acids and trigylcerides.

Lipolysis: The natural process of burning fat for energy. Fat can come from dietary sources or body fat.

Lipolysis testing strips: Also known as LTS. Chemically treated paper test strips or sticks that give a reading when exposed to urine. If acetone is present in the urine as a result of incomplete breakdown of fatty acids and amino acids in the body, the test strips change color, indicating ketosis. This happens when ketone bodies form as a result of a low carbohydrate dietary regimen, allowing fats and proteins to be oxidized (burned) for fuel.

Liver: A large glandular organ, located in the upper abdominal cavity, which secretes bile and is essential to metabolic processes.

Low blood sugar: See **hypoglycemia**.

M

Maltitol: This sugar alcohol is used by food manufacturers as a replacement for carbohydrates such as sucrose. It contributes only 2.1 calories per gram as compared to sucrose's 4 calories per gram; nor does it raise blood glucose as sucrose does.

Metabolic advantage: The benefit gained by switching the body from a glucose metabolism to a fat metabolism, thereby allowing the consumption of a greater number of calories than is possible on low fat weight-control programs.

Metabolic resistance: A state in which it is extremely difficult to lose weight, despite restricted dietary consumption.

Metabolism: The process by which foods are transformed into basic elements that can be utilized by the body for energy or growth; the sum of all chemical reactions that go on in living cells. Metabolism includes all the reactions by which the body obtains and spends all the calories it gets from food.

Mineral: In nutrition, a compound nutrient that contains an inorganic substance, such as a metal or other trace element found in the earth's crust. For example, sodium chloride (table salt) is a compound of sodium and chlorine. Minerals play a vital role in regulating many of the body's functions.

Monounsaturated fat: A fatty acid with only one double or triple bond per molecule, it is found in such foods as fowl, almonds, pecans, cashew nuts, peanuts, avocado and olive and canola oil.

N

Net Carbs: The carbohydrates that can be digested and processed by the body as dietary carbohydrate and therefore directly impact blood sugar. The figure for Net Carbs represents the total grams of carbohydrate minus grams of fiber, glycerine and sugar alcohols. Net Carbs are the only carbs that you need to count when you do Atkins.

Nutrient density: A measure of the nutrients a food provides relative to the calories it dispenses. The more nutrients and the fewer calories, the higher its nutrient density.

O

Obesity: An abnormal increase in the proportion of fat cells (as opposed to lean body mass) in the tissues of the body. An individual is considered obese when weight is 20 percent (25 percent in women) or more over the maximum desirable for his/her height. When the excess weight begins to interfere with vital functions such as breathing, the individual is considered morbidly obese. Obesity will increase the risk for illness and death due to diabetes, stroke, coronary artery disease and kidney and gallbladder disorders. The more overweight an individual, the higher the risk becomes. Obesity has been implicated in increased incidence of some types of cancer.

Ongoing Weight Loss: Also known as OWL. In the Atkins Nutritional Approach™, the dietary phase following the more stringent Induction phase. In this phase, individuals find the most liberal level of carb consumption that allows them to enjoy continued weight loss.

Osteoporosis: A disease of the skeleton leading to increased risk of bone fracture. Normal, strong bone is composed of protein, collagen and calcium. Osteoporosis is characterized by the depletion of both calcium and protein, resulting in brittle bones with lower density.

P

Partially hydrogenated oil: See **hydrogenated oil.**

Phytonutrient: Any potentially healthy food component that comes from a plant and may provide a benefit beyond simple nutrition. Vitamins and minerals also are found in plants, but phytonutrients usually have a more profound effect on the metabolism. One major advantage of phytonutrients is their ability to help prevent cancer and other diseases. Some examples include allyl sulfides in garlic, onions and chives and capsaicin in chili peppers. Phytonutrients are usually present in plants in much smaller amounts than vitamins and minerals.

Plateau: In terms of weight loss, a point at which progress temporarily ceases despite continued adherence to the program. This pause may happen for several reasons. For example, on a controlled carb program, a plateau could be the result of a new medication, illness, stress or reduced activity level. With continued compliance to the program, weight loss will eventually resume.

Polycystic ovary syndrome: Also known as PCOS. One of the most frequent causes of female infertility, PCOS is a complex endocrine disorder associated with hormonal imbalance and long-term failure to ovulate. PCOS is characterized by formation of cysts in the ovaries as a result of the failure of the ovary to release an egg. In most cases, the ovaries become enlarged. The disorder afflicts up to 22 percent of women during their childbearing years, although only 10 percent of these women will develop symptoms.

Polyunsaturated fat: Technically, a type of fatty acid with more than one double or triple bond per molecule,

PUFAs are found in fish, corn, walnuts, sunflower seeds, soybeans and cottonseed and safflower oils.

Potassium: A mineral necessary for muscle building, normal body growth and glycogen formation, potassium assists in protein synthesis from amino acids and in carbohydrate metabolism. Fish such as salmon, cod, flounder and sardines are good sources of potassium. Various other types of meats also contain potassium. Vegetables including broccoli, peas, lima beans, tomatoes, potatoes (especially their skins) and leafy green vegetables such as spinach, lettuce and parsley contain potassium. Fruits that contain significant sources of potassium are citrus fruits, apples, bananas and apricots (especially dried apricots).

Pre-Maintenance: The third phase of the Atkins Nutritional Approach™, when no more than 10 pounds remain to be lost. In this phase, carbohydrate intake is increased to the point where weight loss is deliberately slowed to a crawl. When goal weight has been sustained for at least a month, the individual then moves on to Lifetime Maintenance.

Processed food: In contrast to whole foods, foods that may contain additives and have often been treated to enhance looks, taste or shelf life. Nutrients are often added to replace those destroyed by processing.

Protein: One of three macronutrients that provide calories. Protein, needed for the growth and repair of all human tissues, is composed of approximately 20 amino acids. The body can make 13 of them; the other 9, called essential amino acids, must be obtained in the diet. Protein provides the body with energy and heat, and is needed for the manufacture of hormones, antibodies and enzymes. It also maintains the body's acid/alkali balance.

Psyllium husk: The seed coating of a soluble plant-based fiber. In combination with adequate water intake, it adds bulk to the stool, promoting regularity. Soluble fiber has also been shown to help lower blood cholesterol levels.

R

Refined carbohydrate(s): Plant foods that have undergone a process by which their coarse parts are removed. For example, when wheat is refined into flour, the bran, germ and husk, all healthful components rich in vitamins or fiber, are taken away.

S

Saturated fat: A type of fatty acid found in meat, egg yolks, dairy products and fish, as well as coconut and palm oils. Saturated fats are generally solid at room temperature.

Starch: A plant polysaccharide composed of thousands of small sugar molecules. Sources of starch include grains, legumes and vegetables such as potatoes and beets. Starches are used as thickening agents in many products such as bread, cakes and pasta.

Stroke: A group of brain disorders that occur when the blood supply to any part of the brain is interrupted. The brain requires about 20 percent of the circulation of blood in the body. Even a brief interruption to the blood flow can cause decreases in brain function. Symptoms vary with the area of the brain affected and commonly include such problems as changes in vision or speech, decreased movement or sensation in a part of the body or changes in the level of consciousness. If the blood flow is decreased for longer than a few seconds, brain cells in the area are destroyed, causing permanent damage to that area of the brain or even death.

Sucralose: An artificial sweetener made from sugar that tastes 600 times as sweet as sugar and provides 0 calories per gram.

Sucrose: See **sugar**.

Sugar: A disaccharide composed of glucose and fructose. It is commonly known as table sugar, beet sugar or cane sugar. Sugar also occurs in many fruits and some vegetables and grains.

Sugar alcohols: Also known as polyols, sugar alcohols are sugar molecules with hydroxy, or alcohol, groups attached. Sugar alcohols have many of the characteristics of carbohydrates, such as bulking and sweetening, but provide fewer calories, and do not impact blood glucose as sugar does.

Systolic blood pressure: The maximum blood pressure, which occurs during contraction of the left ventricle of the heart chamber. It is the higher number in a blood pressure reading, expressed as the higher part, or numerator, of the fraction. When you say your blood pressure is 110 over 70, 110 is the systolic blood pressure.

T

Thermogenesis: A process that generates heat, especially in the body.

Trans fatty acids: Also known as trans fats, fats that have been altered to a form that the body cannot digest. Examples include hydrogenated and partially hydrogenated oils created by a manufacturing process as well as fats that have been exposed to excessive heat by cooking. See also **hydrogenated oils**.

Triglyceride: The chief form of fat in the diet and the major storage form of fat in the body. Serum levels of triglycerides indicate how much fat is moving through or clogging arteries. A level below 150 milligrams per deciliter (mg/dl) is considered healthy.

Type 1 diabetes: Insulin-dependent diabetes is a less common type of diabetes than Type 2, in which insufficient or no insulin is produced, requiring daily injections of insulin. Juvenile-onset diabetes, an auto-immune condition, is more likely to be Type 1. It is a life-long condition requiring the use of insulin.

Type 2 diabetes: Also known as non-insulin-dependent diabetes, this is the more common type of diabetes. The body's fat cells resist the action of insulin, resulting in the inability to burn up the blood sugar (that comes from dietary carbohydrates), resulting in more sugar circulating in the bloodstream.

U

Uric acid: A form of nitrogenous waste, uric acid is an odorless compound formed in the body as a result of protein metabolism. It is present in small amounts in human urine; high levels can result in kidney stones and gout.

V

Vitamin: An organic nutrient (as opposed to a mineral, which is inorganic) essential for normal physiological and metabolic functions of the body. Most vitamins cannot be synthesized by the body and must be obtained from food or supplements.

W

Weight training: Also known as resistance training, this is the use of free weights or weight machines to provide resistance for developing muscle strength and endurance. A person's own body weight may also be used to provide resistance in the case of sit-ups, pull-ups or abdominal crunches.

White flour: The finely ground endosperm of the wheat seed, this flour has been refined for maximum softness and whiteness. It also may be bleached. The bran, a source of fiber, and germ have both been removed.

White sugar: Pure sucrose or table sugar that is produced by dissolving and concentrating crystals of sucrose or dextrose so that it recrystallizes.

➤ The Science Behind Atkins

➤ Research That Validates Low Carbohydrate Weight Loss

Controlled carbohydrate nutritional practices are now more than ever being studied for efficacy and long-term safety as well as in connection with a variety of health and disease modalities. Certain studies are specifically focused on the outcomes that result from following the Atkins Nutritional Approach™ (ANA); others look at similar controlled carbohydrate protocols. The following 15 studies were among the most recently published (or presented) when this book went to press. You can find the complete library of published studies in The Science Behind Atkins, at *www.atkins.com*.

Brehm, B. J., Seeley, R. J., Daniels, S. R., et al., "A Randomized Trial Comparing a Very Low Carbohydrate Diet and a Calorie-Restricted Low Fat Diet on Body Weight and Cardiovascular Risk Factors in Healthy Women," *The Journal of Clinical Endocrinology and Metabolism*, 88(4), 2003, pages 1617–1623.

Foster, G. D., Wyatt, H. R., Hill, J. O., et al., "A Randomized Trial of a Low-Carbohydrate Diet for Obesity," *The New England Journal of Medicine*, 348(21), 2003, pages 2082–2090.

Greene, P., Willett, W., Devecis, J., et al., "Pilot 12-Week Feeding Weight-Loss Comparison: Low-Fat vs Low-Carbohydrate (Ketogenic) Diets." Abstract presented at The North American Association for the Study of Obesity Annual Meeting 2003, *Obesity Research,* 11S, 2003, page 95OR.

Hays, J. H., Gorman, R. T., Shakir, K. M., "Results of Use of Metformin and Replacement of Starch With Saturated Fat in Diets of Patients With Type 2 Diabetes," *Endocrinology Practice*, 8(3), 2002, pages 177–183.

Hickey, J., Hickey, L., Heritage Medical Center Partners, Hilton Head, S. C.; Hepburn, J., Yancy, W., Westman, E. C., Duke University, Durham, N. C., "Treating the Metabolic Syndrome with Carbohydrate Restriction." Abstract presented at Nutrition Week 2003, American Society of Parenteral and Enteral Nutrition.

O'Brien, K. D., Brehm, B. J., Seeley, R. J., "Greater Reduction in Inflammatory Markers with a Low Carbohydrate Diet than with a Calorically Matched Low Fat Diet." Presented at American Heart Association's Scientific Sessions 2002 on Tuesday, November 19, 2002, Abstract ID: 117597.

Samaha, F. F., Iqbal, N., Seshadri, P., et al., "A Low-Carbohydrate as Compared with a Low-Fat Diet in Severe

Obesity," *The New England Journal of Medicine,* 348(21), 2003, pages 2074–2081.

Sharman, M. J., Kraemer, W. J., Love, D. M., et al., "A Ketogenic Diet Favorably Affects Serum Biomarkers for Cardiovascular Disease in Normal-Weight Men," *The Journal of Nutrition,* 132(7), 2002, pages 1879–1885.

Sondike, S. B., Copperman, N., Jacobson, M. S., "Effects of a Low-Carbohydrate Diet on Weight Loss and Cardio-vascular Risk Factor in Overweight Adolescents," *The Journal of Pediatrics,* 142(3), 2003, pages 253–258.

Stadler, D. D., Burden, V., Connor, W., et al., "Impact of 42-Day Atkins Diet and Energy-Matched Low-Fat Diet on Weight and Anthropometric Indices," *FASEB Journal,* 17(4–5). Abstract of the 12th Annual FASEB Meeting on Experimental Biology: Translating the Genome; Abstract ID: 453.3, San Diego, CA, April 11–15, 2003.

Volek, J. S., Gómez, A. L., Kraemer, W. J., "Fasting Lipoprotein and Postprandial Triacylglycerol Responses to a Low-Carbohydrate Diet Supplemented with N-3 Fatty Acids," *Journal of the American College of Nutrition,* 19(3), 2000, pages 383–391.

Volek, J. S., Sharman, M. J., Gómez, A. L., et al., "An Isoenergetic Very Low Carbohydrate Diet Improves Serum HDL Cholesterol and Triacylglycerol Concentrations, the Total Cholesterol to HDL Cholesterol Ratio and Postpran-dial Lipemic Responses Compared with a Low Fat Diet in Normal Weight, Normolipidemic Women," *The Journal of Nutrition,* 133(9), 2003, pages 2756–2761.

Volek, J. S., Sharman, M. J., Love, D. M., et al., "Body Composition and Hormonal Responses to a Carbohydrate Restricted Diet," *Metabolism*, 51(7), 2002, pages 846–870.

Volek, V. S., Westman, E. C., "Very-Low-Carbohydrate Weight-Loss Diet Revisited," *Cleveland Clinic Journal of Medicine*, 69(11), 2002, pages 849–862.

Westman, E. C., Yancy, W. S., Edman, J. S., et al., "Effect of 6-Month Adherence to a Very Low Carbohydrate Diet Program," *The American Journal of Medicine*, 113(1), 2002, pages 30–36.

Lose Weight, Feel Great, *and* Save Money Too!
Get $1.00 off when you purchase

DR. ATKINS' NEW DIET REVOLUTION

The Must-Have NEW Edition

The world's #1 diet and complementary medicine expert updated his program for a new audience—offering new information based on controlled carbohydrate principles. It includes:

- All you need to know in order to achieve permanent weight loss and a lifetime of well-being
- New controlled carbohydrate recipes for delicious breakfasts, lunches, dinners, snacks and desserts
- The very latest in scientific research
- And much, much more!

Buy and enjoy *Dr. Atkins' New Diet Revolution* (available now), then send the coupon below along with your proof of purchase for *Dr. Atkins' New Diet Revolution* to Avon Books, and we'll send you a check for $1.00.

Mail receipt and coupon for *Dr. Atkins New Diet Revolution* (0-06-001203-X) to:
AVON BOOKS/HarperCollins*Publishers* Inc.
P.O. Box 767, Dresden, TN 38225

NAME _____

ADDRESS _____

CITY _____

STATE/ZIP _____
*Offer valid only for residents of the United States and Canada. Offer expires 4/1/04.

ATR 0104

Get healthy the Atkins way!

Two must-have companions for better living.

THE ATKINS SHOPPING GUIDE
0-06-072200-2
$7.50 ($9.99 Can.)

THE HANDY POCKET COMPANION TO THE #1 NEW YORK TIMES BESTSELLER, *DR. ATKINS' NEW DIET REVOLUTION*

ATKINS HEALTH & MEDICAL INFORMATION SERVICES

• Indispensable tips and guidelines for successfully stocking your low carb kitchen
• What to buy and what to avoid
• The ideal supermarket carry-along
• How to read and understand food labels

Coming soon

Atkins Diabetes Revolution
0-06-054008-7
$25.95 ($36.95 Can.)

#1 New York Times Bestselling Author

THE GROUNDBREAKING APPROACH TO PREVENTING AND CONTROLLING DIABETES

Atkins Diabetes Revolution

ROBERT C. ATKINS, M.D.

THERE'S NOTHING TO EAT ON ATKINS® EXCEPT...

Advantage
bars and shakes

Almond Brownie Bar
Chocolate Peanut
Butter Bar
Café au Lait Shake
Vanilla Shake

Crunchers
snack chips

Original Chips
Nacho Chips
BBQ Chips
Sour Cream & Onion
Chips

Quick Cuisine
mixes and pastas

Corn Muffin Mix
Pancake/Waffle Mix
Elbows & Cheese Pasta Side
Fettuccine Alfredo Pasta Side

Supplements
vitamins and minerals

Accel
Basic #3
Dieter's Advantage
Essential Oils

Morning Start
breakfast foods

Cinnamon Bun Bar
Apple Crisp Bar
Banana Nut Harvest Cereal
Crunchy Almond Crisp Cereal

Indulge
chocolate candy

Peanut Butter Cups
Chocolate Mint Wafer
Caramel Nut Chew
Almond Bar

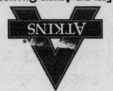

ATKINS

FEEL THE ATKINS CHANGE™

Look for the red "A℠" to find controlled-carb
products where healthy foods are sold.

www.atkins.com